TOUWA
—————— AND ——————
THE DUSTY ROAD TRAVELLED

TOUWA
—— AND ——
THE DUSTY ROAD TRAVELLED

A family story through a generation followed during the life of Touwa

[handwritten signature]
30/11/12

To Shukria

Dr. P V Mroso

authorHOUSE®

AuthorHouse™
1663 Liberty Drive
Bloomington, IN 47403
www.authorhouse.com
Phone: 1-800-839-8640

Published by AuthorHouse   10/18/2012

ISBN: 978-1-4772-3767-0 (sc)
ISBN: 978-1-4772-3768-7 (e)

CONTENTS

Acknowledgements

To my wife Dora, children Heidi, Anthony, Steven and grandchildren (listed in the book)who will have many questions answered.

To my Sister Mkaleso (Theresa)
To my brothers Ndesumbuka (Mathew), Melikoi (Francis), Tabu (Daniel)and Tabuni (Tadei)including uncle Katarimo, cousin Mtele (Oswald)who collectively contributed to some of the contents of this book.

For their friendship and support tribute is given to all other 15 brothers and sisters

To all those family members who have passed on.

Preface

Dr Paul V Mroso (BSc, PhD, MGPhC)was born in Nanjara. He owes his progress from the encouragement given by Shenji (Kahumba Nakovisi Silayo)his beloved grandad and his father Salema (Vincent Salema Kimario)who worked hard to pay the costs of education, with added help from scholarships granted by the Government of Tanzania and WHO (World Health Organisation). As a Pharmacy graduate he returned home to work at Keko Pharmaceutical Plant where he was the Production department leader until he returned to Aston University for a Ph D in Pharmaceutical Sciences.After graduation, circumstances beyond his control led to a request of a UK residency for him and his family. The years that followed Paul worked as a community Pharmacist. He took many holidays to visit his family at Nanjara and as the years passed he started to visit Illasit, Moshi and Dar es Salaam as some of the family moved away from Nanjara.

INTRODUCTION TO CHAPTER 1

Life at the foot of Kilimanjaro

The early days:

Sitting down in front of his hut one evening, admiring and enjoying the beautiful sunset over the Kilimanjaro, as many before him had done and feeling the cool fresh wind from the mountain blowing over the banana plants, Shenji received a message that the *'Mangi'* wanted to see him in the morning.

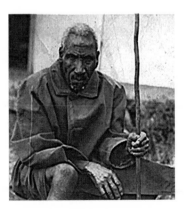

Shenji at age 100

In normal circumstances he would witness the full sunset, hear the last call of many birds as they settle in their nests, and enjoy the hissing noises of the tropical insects as darkness starts. He would even hear the flapping soothing noise made by the banana leaves in the wind and the singing and hissing of the cypress trees and the noise made by the bush that appear to try to stop the wind.

That moment however was far from normal as it was not normal for the great ruler of the community, the Great Chief that was *'Mangi'* to send a message requiring ones attendance the next day. The norm was that he would be called to attend at an instant. Secondly the message was not delivered by a law enforcement man but with respect and courtesy, by one of the many junior chiefs who usually ruled on behalf of the great Chief, *'Mangi'*. Shenji was a prominent man in the community, well known and respected as he had a small heard of cattle and other livestock, he delivered 'Mangi's' dues like taxes paid in promptness. The taxes were paid in large pieces of meat whenever he slaughtered an animal, which was not often as he was not rich and an unmarried man. He thought deeply to see if there was anything he had done, well or bad that required *'Mangi's'* attention. He could not think of any problem, so he proceeded into his hut start to roast on a log fire a succulent piece of steak from a slaughtered cow given by a friend, earlier in the day. With a glass of fermented milk and roast banana to supplement his steak, Shenji's dinner was complete and he proceeded to sleep.

The thought of meeting *'Mangi'* in the morning interrupted his sleep. Early in the morning he asked his helpers to take the animals to pasture while he spruced himself in preparation to meet 'Mangi'. He wore his heavy long mackintosh, his animal hide shoes and his hat. He did not wrap himself with a blanket as most folks did as his mackintosh kept him warm in the cool air of Kilimanjaro.

The journey was by walking, taking at least half an hour through the local community streets that linked hut to hut, dwelling to dwelling, village to village. The streets were footpaths made by many feet walking over the same route year after year. The paths were between bananas, fruit trees, hedges, farm plots and hard wood trees. The paths were not straight; they meandered to avoid any obstacles, making a distance of a kilometre appear as three kilometres. The advantage of such paths was that they are very narrow and fully protected the travellers from the strong suns rays by the tall overgrowth of trees and shrubs that were the feature of the land at the foot of Kilimanjaro.

On arrival at the 'Mangi's place Shenji was surprised to see many other ordinary people he knew in the village. These were people who always met Shenji during their socializing events. Since they knew one another, they quietly asked if one knew the purpose of the meeting. The twenty people were not the powerful junior chiefs, the rich merchants, or the highly educated, but simple folk who had one thing in common. They were the real villagers who had hardly left their villages, had few animals, cattle, sheep and goats an added problem of little land for grazing. They knew they had done nothing wrong because if that was the case they would be called in one by one. After lengthy deliberations on the reasons for the invitation, they concluded that the talk was of some good issue. Before they relaxed too much, one of the '*Mangi's* attendants indicated to all the invitees to go into the inner courtyard where it was private to talk to '*Mangi*'. Inside the Mangi's courtyard all went silent in respect of the Great Chief. A big man wearing a big warm coat, shoes, a hat and over his shoulders hung a nicely decorated blanket with red and yellow stripes, came our as two huge doors were opened. All in the courtyard bowed and shouted in unison: *"hai Mangi Ang'anyi"* meaning greetings great (big)Chief. The *Mangi*, whose name was Yohani Matolo, gave a sign for all to sit down. Every one found a bench, a stone, a folding chair, a fallen banana stem or a stool to sit on. It was after they were all seated that the *'Mangi'* started to speak.

"My friends, you all know that you all pay your taxes to me well whenever you kill your livestock or when you harvest crops I get my share. You know all of you make the best 'mbege' except Shenji who is not married." At that stage all laughed and muttered some comments. 'Mbege' was the local alcoholic beverage made from boiled ripe bananas and flavoured with malt made from millet. *"You see my friends",* the *'Mangi'* continued, *"Shenji has a small herd of cattle but enough to pay a dowry for a wife who will help him make good 'mbege'. Where I was asking you to go there will be more green pastures for your livestock."* On hearing that Shenji's eyes opened wide in anticipation of the new pastures and could not resist standing up and asking a question or rather to compliment his Chief. Shenji stood up and when *Mangi* allowed him to talk he said: *"hai Mangi Ang'anyi,* I will marry as soon as I see the new pastures and will bring you the best *'mbege'*. They all laughed and the *'Mangi'* took the opportunity to be serious and started the agenda of the meeting in earnest. The *'Mangi'* resumed: *"I have called you here to ask you to do a tough job. It involves going away from the village to lands ten to twenty kilometres from here to take bigger lands for yourselves and your friends, to get bigger green pastures and settle there. You have heard the land around river Tarakea and beyond to Rongai, that is the land!"* Thinking of their livestock and the bigger pastures all the men overcame their fears of bandits,

wild animals and the unknown dangers and unanimously promised the Mangi that they were willing to go. It was a triumphant success to *'Mangi Ang'anyi'* who had planned to send groups of twenty people at a time for strength and security. He did not tell his subjects the strategy as that would probably scare them. The real reason was that in the nearby country Europeans had shown an appetite to the fertile lands on the slopes of Mount Kenya and the Mangi in his wisdom could prevent such encroachment to his lands by distributing his people sparsely to ensure most of the good land was occupied, as the foot of Mount Kilimanjaro was the most obvious European land grab destination. Mangi was also pleased with the response and he promised ten heads of cattle to anyone who settled in the new land. He concluded the meeting by giving the twenty men the plan of action and the day of departure which was the next day due to the urgency of the matter. The Mangi wanted to be first in the race for the Tarakea land. Shenji's group of twenty was the vanguard team, in the rush to occupy the whole area of Tarakea on the slopes of Mount Kilimanjaro.

Shenji's name was uttered by the Mangi. That made him an instant leader. He was expected to lead the first delegation to conquer the bush of Tarakea and colonise it. A meeting was held immediately after the 'Mangi' had left and agreed on time to leave. That evening the spears and machetes were sharpened, extra weapons like bow and arrows were assembled, food, water, and a few livestock to provide food on arrival or on the travel as the need arose were selected.

The twenty men started early to walk northwards towards the Tarakea River through a thick virgin bush full of sharp thorns, sharp grass blades, itching plants and an array of wild animals. Among the animals were the carnivores like the lions and hyenas that could attack humans. The monkeys that were not dangerous could steal their food while the birds gave an alert when there was activity in the bush. The men used the tip of the mountain in the west as a compass marker, to help them to navigate northwards. There were small animals that could be hunted to provide food. After twelve hours of walking in the bush, while making their own footpath, they were half way to river Tarakea which was recognised as the river with very deep gorges and very difficult to cross. At night it was too dark to walk they made a camp fire on an area where they felt safe. They slept in shifts to avoid being eaten. Those who were awake could hear the jungle songs made by lions, hyenas, elephants, buffaloes, monkeys with the chorus from jungle insects that hissed and sometimes fly about emitting light. The most annoying sound of the jungle was the laughing hyenas especially when hunting and during a catch and eating. When they walk up in the morning all were alive, thanked their Sun God 'Ruwa', and continued their exploratory journey. The vanguard group led by Shenji made makers in order to speed up the return journey and subsequent outward trips. The markers included tree branch cutting, hanging of a cow horn or a calabash on a tall tree, tree bark stripping and making note of the huge trees. As they approached the Tarakea River, the land was gradually composed of grassland type of vegetation in comparison to the bush they had to cross. At Tarakea river area, one could see far distances, unlike the bushy thicket type of vegetation that was crossed. When they made a glimpse of the Tarakea River, the crystal clear water, the deep gorge that was not easy to cross that offered protection from the north made that new land look like a paradise on earth. They imagined the use of the tall grass to make shacks that could later be improved into huts. They unanimously agreed to settle. They built one hut at a time in co-operation and soon twenty huts were built. The men surveyed the land, noted a large tropical wood forest in the west directly below the mountain, water in the river and an ample supply of grass to build huts and forage for the livestock. With the determination to stay, a meeting was held to apportion the land for individual and for community purposes. With a hut built as the base, ten of the travellers were sent back to report to the Mangi, then to return with wives, livestock, corn, banana seed plants, and bean seeds including those of millet.

The making of a village:

When the wives arrived, they were followed by children and a village was on the making. Shenji had to keep the promise he made to the Mangi that was to marry after seeing the green pastures. He returned to Mangi with a wife, Yohana Mamnana, to request his promised ten heads of cattle to drive to his new settlement. The new settlement was full of people; the number was close to a hundred. That number included the twenty vanguards, their wives, the children and other dependents and helpers. The settlement was becoming a village with farms of bananas and other food crops with lots of livestock. As the Mangi dispatched more groups some crossed the Tarakea River and eventually the Tarakea area had more than a hundred villages that had to have names and Shenji's settlement became known as Nanjara Village. Nanjara meant wilderness.

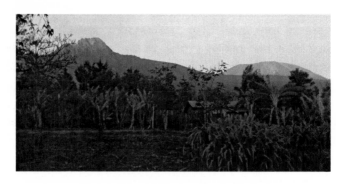

Spectra view Kilimanjaro at sunrise

*The village of Nanjara today and the colourful mountain
Kilimanjaro as viewed by Shenji's Group on a cloudless
morning sunrise*

The village stretched along the south side of river
Tarakea bordered by the thick wood tree tropical forest to
the west and extended almost to the border with Kenya to
the east and to a small stream called Msangai to the south.
News of ample food crops like beans and maize, made
migration so fast that Mangi's persuasion was no longer
necessary. It was the greatest economic growth period that
led to the establishment of markets to sell and exchange
produce and livestock. Mangi and his junior chiefs he had
appointed became rich from the taxes. The people started to
relax and enjoy the fruits of their labour that the fertile land
provided. The drinking of 'mbege' and roast meat eating
with boiled or roast bananas was the best style in which
Chagga people conducted their business. They relaxed,
celebrated or even conducted funerals in the same manner.
They turned many occasions like in courtship, marriages,
child birth and even in mourning into a drinking and
eating occasions. In courtship for example, goats or even

cows were slaughtered each time the two parties met to discuss dowry, and such meetings were not counted on one hand. Childbirth was a period of celebrating and singing songs of praise to the man and the healthy woman who gave birth. A song was usually sung after a consumption of a good amount of 'mbege' whose chorus was: *"hauyese ngalya ngayuta, hauyese ngalya ngalemwa"*. The chorus was repeated after a praising comment like *'the maker of this mbege is the best in all he does'*. The chorus would then mean *'go back again as we have eaten to the full and can eat no more'*, but they do not say what was to be done. The hidden meaning was "to do it again to get another child to enable us to celebrate". The songs of the Chagga have all the same basic theme of praise with a message that was hidden such that children would not decipher. When there was a dispute between neighbours, man and his wife or brothers, no Chagga courts (meaning the assembly of elders)would even consider listening without an offer of 'mbege'. 'Mbege' was the pivot of Chagga society.

The other side of the Chagga people was their hard working ethics. The party food in so many celebrations was a result of hard work.

The happy and hard working Chagga:

Early in the morning it was working up to eat a small breakfast usually fermented milk with a roast banana, next to cut and fetch grass for animals kept inside the huts in a bid to fatten then in excess for lard which had many uses. Taking the large herd of cattle, goats and sheep to the pastures was the next task that was done in rotation by the villagers. Farming work dominated the activity in most days.

There was an existence of a highly organised community service that ensured that all could eat, gain property and build their huts. The village co-operated in building one person a hut and the rotation went on until every person had a decent hut. Farming was also a co–operative work usually by the women although the task of a new farm from bush was a man's work. Wood chopping was duty for older boys while the younger boys' duty would be to run with the chicken to catch it for dinner. That was when they could spare some time from their technical work of building carts, wheelbarrows and bicycled from wood, lubricating the wheels with lard. Laughing and giggling, the girls on their way to the stream to fetch water have pots, guards or cooking pans balanced on their heads. The water fetching duty for the girls looked like an unworthy task but it provided the girls with a social platform where they meet and talk more freely away from their mothers The adolescent boys knew some strategic places to meet in order to observe the girls, they unwittingly however thought that the girls did not know. It was at those times that the boys ready to marry would start their advances. A boy would ask a little girl to tell an older mature girl that the boy wanted to talk and that was for serious relationship. That style of contact could be in persistence for a while until the girl agrees to talk to the boy. When the message was rude, however, a little boy would be sent to tell a mature girl that the man said to go to collect the banana as it is ripe. That kind of message would not be sent again to the same girl or by the same boy, because the little boy would get a slap from the girl. It was a rude massage of a sexual undertone.

Chagga marriages: the old, the express and the modern:

Very early in the formation of the Chagga culture, those were the days when animal hide was used as clothing, beads as the jewellery of the day and skin moisturizer was based on animal oil in the form of lard or the rubbing on the skin the basic raw animal fat. It was the days that wars were being fought, and the treasured capture were women for procreation and livestock for wealth. As the wars diminished and prosperity reigned, certain habits and behaviours acquired during the warring years were incorporated in the culture of the newly formed communities that were living at peace. The old system of acquiring a wife was a rather harsh process measured at today's standards, as described by Touwa's uncle Musee son of Katarimo

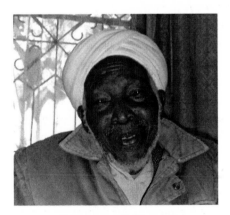

Musee son of Katarimo

When boys start to show the signs of manhood, parents used to think and work hard for the boy to find a suitable wife. It was not a simple job; frantic activities were in motion, first to ensure the boy was interested in acquiring a wife. Second was to search for a suitable family with girls ready for marriage. It was after identifying such a family that the drama started. For a family to be deemed suitable there were a number of secretly conducted checks more intense that the current CRB (*Criminal Records Bureau*) checks carried out in the UK:

- A family of the girl was to have no close relation to the boy's family
- A family was to have no hereditary diseases, the most notable one in memory was epilepsy locally known as '*kifafa*', a condition that was least understood and greatly feared.
- A family was not extravagant to an extent of striping their assets to poverty and possibly showing signs of vagrancy.

Finally, a family that lacks ambition, direction or progress even when opportunities were in place for riches was also disallowed. That condition was thought to be due to a '*curse*' that hampered their opportunity to fortunes.

In addition to all those checks there was a game of luck that was asking 'Ruwa' the great God of the Chagga, to give guidance. A number of elders, not less than three would attempt to read a leaf from an '*ilaka*' (*an evergreen bush revered as a sign of the Chagga as it is believed that where that bush grows a Chagga person can live*)bush as some people may read a palm. When the majority agree that the marriage would be a success, the next step of talking to the girl's family started. At that stage the girl's family does the essential secret checks and rituals on the boy's family. A positive outcome means a marriage may take place.

The mother of the young man intended to marry will meet with the girl's mother to ask her to accept the marriage of their children. There could be a refusal at that stage but it was not the norm. When a marriage was agreed, the boy would introduce the girl to his friends as the girl he intends to marry. At that stage there was another hurdle and that was another boy may also be interested in acquiring that girls as a wife or talk to the girl with that possibility of switching. That fear made it necessary to speed matters after the introduction. Quick plans are made to snatch the girl, carry her to the boy's hut and perform a ritual of making the girl into submission to her man. The ritual that involved good humour was to tie one leg from knee to the toes with beads and strings to ensure that she can't run fast or possibly she can't cross her legs too tightly. The next morning the two mothers would be keen to ensure the sexual state of the daughter. A virgin gave pride to the girl's mother, who would have a reputation of looking after her girls well. In the event she was no virgin, unfavourable rumours would emerge but usually the marriage would continue. It was after three days of pampering, rubbed with oils to ensure the skin shines and good feeding that made a Chagga marriage, when the girl would come out of the hut and be welcome to her new family. That was when 'mbege' drinking, meat eating and possible lots of singing take place to celebrate the marriage.

With time, wealth increased, but its distribution brought about the divisions of the rich and the poor that influenced attitudes toward marriages. There were refusals of marriages based on wealth. Some families did not accept that state of affairs and that led to express marriage styles that had roots of love. The express marriage system that avoided parental involvement was cheap and did break the wealth barrier, but of course there were dangers as the essential checks were not scrutinised.

In the event the girl who got a polite message likes the man a meeting would take place most probably at a friend who had 'mbege'. If by good luck they like one another the boy would suggest marriage and again if that was ok the boy would entice the girls to see his place. After several of such meetings, one of the enticements would be to go to the boy's hut! That time would usually be late at night. If the girl enters the man's hut, the door is shut, and the companions just return home to report where the girl was. That was technically marriage, the ceremony followed later, during that time the girl would reside with the husband. Issues of dowries are settled later but in urgency before children are born. There are occasions when the girl is encouraged by friends who push her into the hut. Once the door is shut it was marriage, the fast track style of acquiring a wife by the not so rich, circumvented all the long expensive betrothal proceedings or courting rituals.

The courtship process, Chagga style of modern marriage preparation is complex, expensive and it is not certain whether one person could remember it all especially when one's daughter is to get married. One has to recall or try to remember the complex process one's father had to take for him to acquire a wife. After the young man who intends to marry informs his father, that he has met a girl who also loves him, parents in both families usually checked secretly for unacceptable issues like suicide in the family, mental problems, and some debilitating diseases like epilepsy *('kifafa')*that were not understood and were frightful. They also checked if there was close family relationship and any bad secrets a family may hide, like abnormalities or unacceptable behaviours like stealing or laziness. The reputation of a family known for its hard working and honesty was a major asset. When that hurdle of secret checking activity is completed, it when betrothal starts.

The father after deliberating with confidants sends two emissaries to the girl's father to inform of the young man's intensions, and to receive an answer from him in order to proceed. When the young mans family had a good personality, passes the vetting process and with wealth measured by the number of cattle in possession, there was usually a swift 'yes'.

Stage two was to invite the parents of the girl to visit and party with the boy's parents. When the term 'parents' was used, it meant all the close friends and their wives from both sets of parents including aunties and uncles and their friends. That was a large party with the significance of introductions as the intended marriage would bring them closer as a family. During that party the issue of dowry would be discussed but not finalised. The party involves the slaughter of a large cow or a number of sheep. That was also to show and impress the visiting family that their daughter was joining a great and not a feeble family. There was usually plenty of eating and drinking with joyful loud singing. The greater the singing the better the party was and greater the satisfaction.

Stage three: the brothers, sisters and cousins from both sides of the two families would party again at the boy's father expense to familiarise with one another. That party of the youngsters would include dancing to music produced by one string instrument, drinking the local brew and eating meat of slaughtered goats. It was during those types of parties of youngsters that other friendships that led to marriages were also forged.

Stage four: there were a series of exchange of presents. Examples of presents included bunches of bananas, millet grain (used to make the local brew), milk in guards, meat when a sheep is slaughtered, and well brewed local brew. During these exchanges, respect and family values are established and date of marriage was then set after a meeting with the elders who finalised the dowry and gave their blessings to the marriage. From that stage the boy would address the girl's father as 'DAD' and similarly the girl would address the boy's father.

The marriage ceremony was conducted in a colourful array of dresses with a showcase attitude of portraying superiority in dressing and attire among the women folk. There was also a carnival atmosphere where singing and dancing were conducted in a friendly but competitive manner between the families of the bride and that of the groom. Drinking and eating roast meat with the couple treated with utmost respect and showered with presents usually of farm products made the ceremony completed.

With occasions like that in occurrence as a matter of frequency life was usually an existence fuelled with happiness.

The arrival of Europeans:

Shenji and friends lived luxuriously, a life of plenty, when wealth creation and marrying an extra wife was the norm, with pride when one had plenty of children. The almost utopia living came to a sudden shock that rocked its foundations. It was when the Europeans arrived in Nanjara.

The Europeans came, but not as land thirsty grabbing giants but as polite, cool and friendly missionaries who claimed to spread the word of a Christian God. The entry of such polite people into the village was a spectre. When a boy herding goats, saw some people who appeared very different from the village folks, run very fast to the village to report to the elders, who were just sitting down to have a mid week drink of 'mbege', the spectre of what he had seen. The boy shouted *"I saw person with no skin, he was as red as a skinned goat, and he was seated on a moving machine that makes a noise like one who had eaten too many beans."* The boy continued, *"And he was with others with skins and all were heading towards the river"*. All the elders some wise, some dunce, some tall, some short, some afraid and some courageous, responded to the unanimous call to defend their land. They gathered all their array of weapons that range from spears to bow and arrows including machetes and sticks. Shenji warned them not to kill them until permission was received from Mangi. They all abandoned their luxurious 'mbege' drinking session and moved cautiously towards the skin-less man as described by the boy. When they saw the moving machine which had stopped as the occupants were looking at the land, they were very afraid as no one had seen such machine. The machine was less significant when the man with no skin was actually seen. The calming fact was that he was accompanied by other Chagga people who spoke in a dialect which was slightly understood. The interpreters managed to communicate that they had Mangi's permission to start a school and a church, so they needed a small piece of land to be given by the people of Nanjara. The acknowledgement of a request and that Mangi new of their arrival removed the possibility of confrontation. Although peace was established, the people gazed at the man with no skin. In all respects he looked odd in comparison to the village folk. He was a short, fat; bald with the little hair that was on his head was all brilliant white. He wore a long white robe that covered most of his legs like a woman' long dress, while on his neck he had a white collar that resembled a goat tied on the neck with banana twine on the way to the market, and tied to his waist a kind of belt that resembled a entwined rope that was similar to the ropes they hung a goat with in the process of slaughtering. A chain hung from his neck, attached to it was a wooden piece on which a man with stretched hand was pinned. When tried to speak in Chagga to greet the people, they replied, surprised that he could speak and above all the dialect. It was that moment when they were convinced he was human. Shenji was relieved that there was no confrontation and he told the interpreters to return after seven days to allow his people to decide on where to build the school. On return the interpreters were more fluent in the local dialect and able to communicate better. A piece of land was allocated for school and the church a distant from the village centre as the people of Nanjara did not want a stranger among them. When that land allocation was completed, a shack was built, that became the school and the centre for the talk about the new God that was led by the man who came to be known as *"a white"* man because of his clothes he wore rather than his looks, because they discovered he had skin that was not as brown as their own. Curiosity led to a large attendance at the start. It was when they heard about the new Christian God. The religion believed in one God that was in agreement with the Chagga god 'Ruwa' who was also the only God. There also no conflict when the preacher talked about sex before marriage as the Chagga enforced that rule. But conflict arose when the preacher talked about one man, one wife.

That rule rocked the basis of man superiority, even Mangi was perturbed. The complexity of the multi-wife culture was solved by some clever compromises that accepted those already married without encouraging new commitments. To cool the conflict a cash crop called coffee was introduced that gave many financial security and schools that taught reading and writing that was accepted as progress. With time conversion to Christianity became almost total, as progress, security and wealth were on the rise. The people of Nanjara experienced great changes in wealth, education, trade, new cultures and road and transport infrastructures. The children of Shenji saw and experienced the changes but it was the grandchildren who enjoyed the benefits of the changes through education as an option to cattle herding and agriculture. Nanjara village was then transformed from bush land to green pastures where Salema, the second child of Shenji was born. Salema's mother Yohana Mamnana was the first of Shenji's three wives. She had three children Mkosi, Salema and a girl Rosalia. It is the life of Salema and his descendents that forms the core of the story that follows.

CHAPTER 1

The early days
in the green pastures of home

Thinking:

Sitting down outside his hut on a smooth stone, worn to smoothness over the years by the many bottoms that sat on it before him, Salema was contemplating over many issues of life whilst enjoying the beautiful sunset over the Mawenzi and Kibo peaks of m o u n t a i n Kilimanjaro, the slopes of which the Chagga people live. The red sun appeared to sink into the space between the two peaks of the

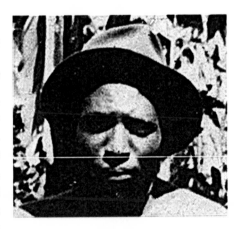

Salema

1

mountain casting a shadow over the slopes bringing the day to an end, and the start of the dark night in a matter of minutes. The stone Salema sat on was known as *'Kijiwe'* meaning a place to think, reflect and plan the future. Salema was in deep thoughts. He had two children Salimu aged five, who was soon to go to school and a girl called Mkaleso aged three. He thought about the school expenses, like uniforms, fees, lunch money and lots more as he heard the older folk talking. He then fully realised that he was a married man with responsibilities, and above all, his wife was expecting, a third child. He also knew that he would need more food that meant to work harder in the farm to cultivate and plant more crops, increase his animal stock, and the feed that would be needed. He thought about tasks that had to be done, like coffee trees, that he had to prune, animals to feed, banana plants that needed constant shaving off dead dry leaves, the removal of overgrowth in the banana plantation, building of a bigger barn for his cattle, or a hut for his expanding family and the list was going on and on, then he switched his thoughts to the needs of the expected new baby.

His thoughts went further to consider the expected child on matters of the animal he had to slaughter on the birthday, the bananas to find to make local brew and even the number of animals he had to put aside for the new child, to cover his or her welfare, including the possible future need of his or her school fees. The good thoughts were those which he had solutions, those made him happy and he could be seen smiling. The worrying thoughts made him look sad. Looking to the sky, Salema enjoyed the constellation of stars that reminded him of Nairobi the big city he had visited when he was a young unmarried man when he was a bachelor. With the exception of the light of the stars, the place was pitch dark every night and frightfully silent except on an occasional barking of a dog, bleating of sheep and goats, a cow mooing or a cat meowing and some pigs could be heard snorting. Chicken could be heard chuckling and from a distance the hooting of an owl or the croaking of a frog. That night however was different as the silence was harrowing, such that even Salema could hear his own heart beat. Despite the weight of responsibility, Salema was optimistically happy as he had solutions to many of the future problems.

He could see some light from his wife's hut, remembering how he built it. It was a round conical structure made entirely by long poles weaved together with smaller flexible poles similar to a basket. Thatching was done using reed grass sewn in with plant fibres from many of the forest plants.

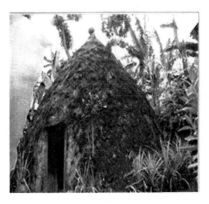

Chagga hut

These huts were prone to fires and termites and had limited lifespan of a decade or two just because the structural poles that anchor the hut were selected from plants that were resistant to water damage and rotting, above all, never eaten by destructive insects like termites. The smoke generated from the log fires used for cooking within the huts imparted a significantly extended life span to six or more decades due to extra protection from the destructive elements like woodlice rot and water damage.

3

Inside the hut were the in-house fed animals like, the milking cow, the male goat the *'horo'* being extra fed and the sheep fattened for the lard, including chickens that visited and slept in as they pleased. Two metres above the floor, was a strong supported ceiling made of wood poles that was used as storage and was also used to place banana bunches

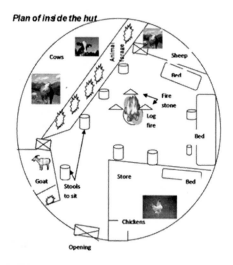

Inside the hut

for a speedy ripening in the process of making the local alcoholic drink called *'mbege'*.

Salema was then 28, five feet seven inches tall, slim, more of a listener than a talker, a confidant to a lot of people as many held him in a high esteem. He was loved in the village because he smiled in response to greetings, he was a hard worker and he organised the community work in the village like weeding of millet crop and building of huts. He was a vanguard in introducing new cash crops like pyrethrum to the village. He was trained in tree planting and he showed many villagers the art and practice of tree planting and explained the future benefits. He had his family respect as he was a loving man. He was however a firm leader but not a bully, talkative but in privacy and never shouted. In public he portrayed shyness by speaking quietly and politely, but in private he was a formidable advisor who gained respect for his wisdom. At his marriage his father had made him fairly wealthy as he then had a heard of about twenty heads of cattle, a number of goats and sheep and a farm that was ten hectors in size, medium in comparison to other plots in those early days. He grew coffee as a cash crop and for food a large area of banana plantation that surrounded the huts. There were also crops like maize, beans, peas, millet, cassava, yams, sweet potatoes and Irish potatoes including fruit trees like lemons oranges, papaya, guava and numerous other seasonal fruits like peppers, berries and pineapples. A hector of his land was filled with all sorts of trees for timber, fire wood, building poles and for fibres. He had one quality of curiosity. He tried but failed to ferment the large crop of lemons from his farm in an attempt to get a beverage. That failure did not deter him from becoming the best *'mbege'* brewer.

The cold August air forced him to go to his wife's hut to eat and get some warmth from the log fire that was always kept burning for cooking and for warmth. Salema never sat too close to the fire, as a matter of respect to his wife. It was good practice for a man to distance himself from the fire to prove that he was strong and could tolerate the cold. Sitting at a distance, Salema had the advantage of looking at his wife with more scrutiny. He saw the beauty, and the gaiety as she cooked and above all the belly which was not small; it was huge, at an advanced stage of pregnancy for the couples' third child.

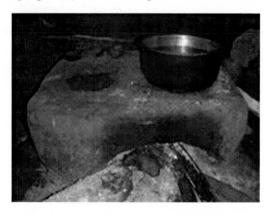

Fire place inside the hut

Salema's thoughts started again, but this time on the day he met his wife, her name, Mkasu a short form of Mkasumaili but she equally answered to the names of Matouwa or Mamroso. She was a fourth child of Touwa's second wife who had one boy, Melikoi and four girls. The four girls were Mamshimbi, Mamkwe, Kandida and Atanasia. Both Salema and Mkasu could not tell when the birth was due; therefore the wise

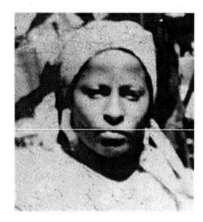

Mkasu on her wedding day

6

thing was to wait. Mkasu, with a smile, asked Salema whether he was ready to eat, but she got no reply as Salema was in deep thoughts of the past and that meant he didn't hear at first, that's why he remarked *'what did you say?'* When he was told again to eat, he signalled to her to wait! He was in deep thoughts, he remembered the day he met Mkasu.

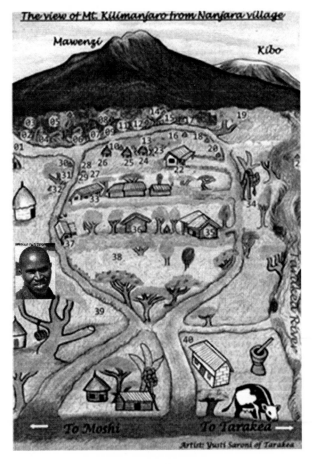

Artist impr of Nanjara

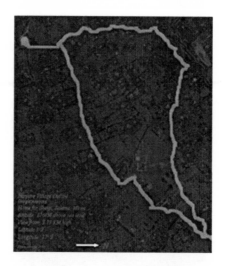

Google view of Nanjara village

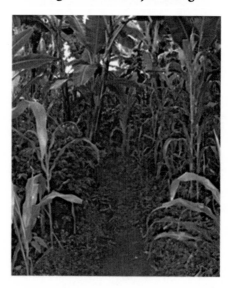

Footpath joining huts

Key: *Names of Residents & Institutions at Nanjara:*

(During the school days of Touwa) 1- "Aulo"** (A meeting place, for collection of livestock to and from pastures)

2—Mdoko

3—Kiberenge

4—Makibonya

5—Karembe

6—Mjeuri

7-Sirikwa

8—Anyika

9-Mmeku

10-Salema

11-Makitushe

12—Makinafu

13—Shenji

14 Mtauli

15-Meriki

16-Yosia (next to his hut was the well**)

17-Kitashinja

18-Msee Machoro (nick—named-Kitengeso)

19—Nursery for the Forestry Department

20-Fidelisi Masika (The husband of Auntie Atanasia)

21-Losina

22-The Dispensary**

23-Manari

24-Marunda

25-Shabani

26-Kahumba

27—Mausa

28—Mamkoku

29—Mtorobo

30-Salekwa

31-Kikari

32-Kimosoyo

33—Nanjara Upper Primary School**

34—The area of great rivalry fights with 'ndulele'**

35—Church **

36-'Kindergarten' (nursery for Nanjara lower primary school**)

37—Nanjara Lower primary school**

38—School playing fields**

39-Matoli

40-Kisumanjia

*Key: Institution or place***

The encounter:

He was travelling from Arusha a town a hundred kilometres away, to see his parents during his annual leave from his job as a forest keeper. He planted and cared for new trees in addition to preserving the natural forest under a supervision of an English gentleman. Travelling home was by foot through forests, fast flowing streams, and even the danger of wild carnivores. That journey which took a total of seven days was taken by a group of young men who survived by eating wild fruits, drinking water from the streams and food from well wishers. At the last eight Kilometres, Salema was alone, as most in the group had arrived at their homes. Salema was not in any danger as he travelled close to habitats. He was very tired, therefore, nothing was of interest to him but to arrive home to Nanjara where his father had started a new farm.

Five kilometres from home, Salema was very tired; he planned to sit down for a little rest just before approaching a small stream that flows with pure crystal clear mountain water. Before he did that however, he noticed a group of girls rushing to the river to fetch water and Salema followed them. May be he wanted water to drink or just to talk to the girls. Salema was twenty, he was a bit shy but the travelling had made him more confident. As he followed the girls he noted one girl that he wanted to talk to, and he thought the best approach was to ask her to use her cup to get some water from the steam for him to drink. Salema said after a little cough, *'may I have a cup of water please as I have travelled from far'.* The girl looked at him, smiled and gave him a calabash full of water. The girl watched Salema drinking the water but before he gave her the calabash back, Salema successfully got to know her name and her father's name, which was Touwa. That name of her father was more important to Salema than that of the girl as it was the father's name that was used at the start of the courtship. Salema started to leave thanking the girl for her kindness, but something strong compelled Salema to

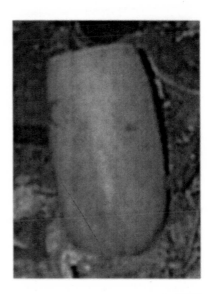

The calabash for drinking mbege

run back to the girl and whispered in her ear: '*I will remember you and soon I will come to take you as my wife to my parents*', then he ran away not waiting for the girl to answer. On remembering that, Salema smiled and looked at his wife Mkasu lovingly. By that time Salema felt that the hut was getting much warmer and needed his food.

Mkasu noticed Salema smiling and asked if he was ready for his dinner. That time he accepted. When Salema was eating, Mkasu had nothing to do but to reminisce about the sweet old days. She remembered the day she gave Salema some water and what he had said, and she had smiled. She also recalled how she had run home fast to give the news to her mother that a boy had said he liked her. She also evoked her memories on the worries she had at that time, like whether the boy was serious, if he was crazy, when he would come if he would be always good and so on, then she remembered her mother's words: '*if you like him you wait*', and she smiled again as her crazy boy was eating the dinner she had just cooked. She glanced at Salema, smiled and felt happy. The thoughts of meeting Mkasu were so sweet that Salema could not stop thinking about the moment his mother was told.

Yohana, Salema's mother, sitting on the stone ('kijiwe') was excited for two reasons. She wanted her boy to stay at home instead of going to the towns where bad things happened to people, and that the Touwa family was a good one, with the added advantage of belonging to the ruling class of junior chiefs. The worry was whether they would allow an unknown boy like Salema to marry into a family of the rulers like Touwa. Shenji, Yohana's husband and Salema's dad, had two distinct sides to his character. He was generous, progressive, kind and loving. The other side of his character was that, he portrayed himself as tough, born leader, no nonsense man with a short temper, very strict and uncompromising, very touchy, and unapproachable as he rarely smiled unlike his son Salema. He had one huge privilege of being a confidant of '*Mangi Ang'anyi*' the big and great chief.

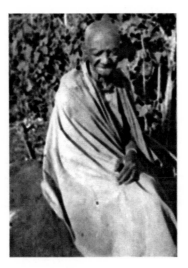

Grandma yohana

Mangi Ang'anyi sent Shenji (pictured sitting on his folding chair and a few other confidants to Tarakea area to colonise the land to prevent Europeans taking over the land. Shenji took a large virgin land mass, bordering the natural forest and the banks of river Tarakea where he could graze and water his large herd of cattle. This land mass was populated and became the village of Nanjara. The Tarakea River provided water and bathing facilities while the forest provided the green pastures to graze the animals and a free source of products like honey, building wood, ropes, thatch grass, fire wood and occasional wild animal meat from hunting. The easy availability of those facilities encouraged a rapid increase in population. The land mass was portioned to families. As time passed the individually owned plots were reduced in size due to subdivision as the families grew bigger, but the huts were built closer to the families for security reasons. Shenji, the originator of Nanjara village, had his friends and family all around him making him feeling very secure. When Shenji arrived home that evening, Yohana called him for a private talk on the boy's possible marriage, and when Touwa's name was mentioned Shenji agreed and when Shenji said 'yes', all that was said was done. Shenji was confident that Touwa could not say no to a confidant of the great chief. Parents in both families usually checked secretly for unacceptable issues like

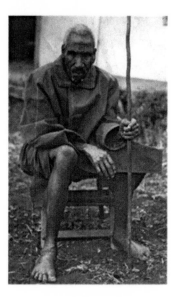

Grandad Shenji

suicide in the family, mental problems, and some debilitating diseases like epilepsy (*'kifafa'*) that were not understood and were frightful. They also checked if there was close family relationship and any bad secrets a family may hide, like abnormalities or unacceptable behaviours like stealing or laziness. The reputation of a family known for its hard working and honesty was a major asset. When Salema was called by his father to be told it was agreed, he was very excited. He remembered how he left early in the morning travelled five kilometres and returning home without his parents realising that he was gone, just to tell Mkasu the news that his parents had agreed and that, news to her father would soon be delivered and how Mkasu ran away signifying pleasure and excitement. With a pause from these thoughts he looked at his wife as he finished eating his dinner and expressed his love and happiness with a smile. He then washed his hands and he bid goodnight to his wife and went to his own hut to sleep. As he left he told his wife to shut the door to show his concerns of her safety.

The courtship process, Chagga style:

In his bed, the thoughts of the past did not diminish therefore he continued to remember the courtship process that was complex and he was not certain whether he could remember it all when his daughter Mkaleso was to get married. He recalled or tried to remember the complex process he or his father had to take for him to acquire a wife. After he informed his father, two emissaries were sent to Touwa to confirm Salema's intentions, and to receive an answer from him in order to proceed. Since Shenji was well known as he had a big personality that matched his large herd of cattle and the best brewer in the village, the answer was a definite 'YES'.

Stage two was to invite the parents of the girl to visit and party with the boy's parents. When the term 'parents' was used, it meant all the close friends and their wives from both sets of parents including aunties and uncles and their friends. That was a large party with the significance of introductions as the intended marriage would bring them closer as a family. During that party the issue of dowry was discussed but not finalised. That party had to involve the slaughter of a large cow or a number of sheep. That was also to show and impress the visiting family that their daughter was joining a great and not a feeble family. There was plenty of eating and drinking with joyful loud singing. The greater the singing the better the party was and greater the satisfaction.

Stage three: the brothers, sisters and cousins from both sides of the two families were invited again at Shenji's residence to party and familiarise with one another. That party of the youngsters included dancing to music produced by one string instrument, drinking the local brew and eating meat of slaughtered goats. It was during those types of parties of youngsters that other friendships that led to marriages were also forged. The proof was that some of Mkasu's sisters were eventually married in the village of Nanjara to husbands who were Salema's friends.

Stage four: there were a series of exchange of presents. Examples of presents included bunches of bananas, millet grain (used to make the local brew), milk in guards, meat when a sheep was slaughtered, and well made local brew. During those exchanges, respect and family values were established and date of marriage was then set after a meeting with the elders who finalised the dowry and gave their blessings to the marriage. From that stage Salema would address Touwa as 'DAD' and Mkasu would do similarly address Shenji. With the knowledge that he remembered most of the complex rituals Salema praised himself with a little giggle and drifted to a smooth baby-like sleep. The marriage styles in the Chagga society had evolved over the years and Salema's thoughts reflected the rituals that were in practice at his early years.

At the marriage ceremony, irrespective of the method used to acquire a wife, there was a colourful array of dresses with a showcase attitude that attempted to portray superiority in dressing and attire among the women folk. The whole affair was in a carnival atmosphere where singing, dancing, drinking and eating roast meat was essential. The couple were treated with utmost respect and were showered with gifts usually of farm products. With occasions like that in occurrence as a matter of frequency life was usually an existence fuelled with happiness.

The neighbours:

The folks of Nanjara that were neighbours to Shenji and Salema during the days when they had young families were happy, friendly, helpful and co-operative. Shenji, Salema's father was the oldest member of the village and as tradition dictated he was respected by all. But Shenji was a leader that ensured he got the respect as those who disobeyed him had their lives made miserable. Most folks addressed one another by the first name but to Salema's recollection no one called Shenji by his first name. There were also some bad people in the village who were jealous of everyone success. They expressed their horrid behaviour by poisoning those who they perceived as getting better than themselves on matters of wealth or children who were progressive. Shenji's children were progressive and so they were targeted. One of Shenji's sons was very ill, and the story was he was poisoned. In normal circumstances no one dared calling names of those they suspected of that behaviour of poisoning, magic or sorcery in the event they might be picked to be harmed. Shenji however, was different. He was a no nonsense leader. He went to *'Aulo'* (a public place of meeting where all livestock was assembled in order to proceed to the forest pastures to feed, returning in the evening where each individual collects their animals) and declared that his neighbour by name as the one who poisoned his son and he challenged him to swear that he did not do! Mako was the name mentioned. Mako did not know what to do because if he was the poison man, he must have been scared as he thought Shenji had a more powerful poison to dare mention his name in public. On the other hand, if he was not the culprit, the mere mention of his name was condemnation. He neither came to 'Aulo' nor showed his face anywhere, even when there was *'mbege'* drinking gathering nearby. Shenji made him a recluse, a punishment similar to a deportation from the village. That was a severe punishment because he would not be able to participate in the closeness spirit. Neighbours would go to one another to borrow items like sugar or salt, some tea leaves, oil to cook or kerosene for the lantern, a match to light a fire or even amber to start a fire. Such punishment would also exclude him from sharing *'mbege'* drinking or getting a portion of honey from the forest. Exclusion of that nature was enough to instil a high level of discipline in the village that promoted happiness, helpfulness and co-operation.

The friendliness went further by generating nick names to match their neighbours' characters. There was for example a *'Kitashinja'* literally mean *'he does not slaughter'* that was a nick name given to a person who was so mean he never slaughters a goat or sheep to give to his neighbours despite enjoying many meat eating periods with them. If ever he had to slaughter, it would be him with his wife to avoid the customary sharing.

There was also a *'Wang'indele'* literally translates as *'they have just sent it to me'*. That was a person who hardly wanted to share freely his *'mbege'*. If a neighbour passed and accidentally find such an individual enjoying a calabash of drink with his wife, he would be told in order to go away with a saying that they do not have any more to give him as that calabash was sent to him not long ago. When closer friends found out about that habit they coined *Wang'indele'* the nick name.

The other nick name indicated wilful character. *'Kisuma njia'* was a nick name of a person who used to dig holes on the walking pathways when people used his land to make a short cut, hence the nick name which translates *to "road digger."*

The younger folk had a *'Kusambie'* which translates to *"wash"* That nick name was given to a light skinned villager who was a teacher, because he was clean and dressed smart relative to the farm workers who were at most times soiled. That nick name however encouraged many to want that nickname by attempting to be cleaner and smarter when they went for *'mbege'* drinking sessions. Nick names originated from looks, characters, the place one lives, behaviour with women or after a drink even those who worked very little or very hard.

Shenji, Salema's dad's name was a nick name that was so entrenched that few people new his really name. That name translates to *'that man who calls everyone a fool'* It was a name given to a strict man whose ways were the only correct ones as he adhered to the protocols of doing things like how to slaughter an animal, how to share and many more Chagga traditions.

'Kitarawa' could be translated as 'the one who bothers people or a tormenter'. If a *'Kitarawa'* wanted something

from you he would come to your place many times like every hour for twelve hours until he gets his wish. A person would be unwise to owe him a 'penny' or a 'farthing' (half of half of a penny).

'Kimbulumbulu' like in Swahili *'mgeugeu'* a person who has a constant excuse to changing his standing on any issue, one can hardly make a pact with *'Kimbulumbulu'*

The level of nicknames may have given birth to real names because the generation that followed may consider a person's nickname as a real name resulting to children having their fathers nickname as their official names.

The meaning of some names may give a clue to situations where nick-names have merged into real individual names. **Salema,** for example means 'when life is tough'. A person born at that time could have that name Salema to remember when life was at the edge of impossibility. **Ndesumbuka** can be described as a period of discomfort, a person born at such time could have that name to signify the state of life at the birth. **Tabu** means hardship, and is a name given to signify such condition. **Tabuni** means in hardship, a period when there was general hardship in the community. There is also **'Kinyeti'** that means *the tail*, signifying a name given to Salema's last child, that may become a real name in the future.

Tarakea, the river:

To Shenji and his companions, the vanguards that discovered Nanjara, saw Tarakea as a mighty river that could not be crossed. In fact Tarakea was a stream whose water was fast flowing with high energy currents from the mountain to the lower more level distant areas of the slopes of Mount Kilimanjaro. The speed and energy of the water curved deep almost vertical gorges that made reaching the water level difficult. The resourceful team that Shenji led made winding paths to overcoming the steep gorges to reach and collect water from the stream. They also dug and made the paths wide to enable the animals to reach the river to drink. The clean, crystal clear water of the river served Shenji's community until the introduction of piped water and man made wells. The strong water currents were able to move large stones from the mountain. The result was smooth river stones and plenty of sand that helped to filter and make the water always clean. The water level in the stream fluctuated greatly with the seasons. The section of the stream where Shenji settled did not dry completely during long periods of dry weather, but the it became a dry bed further eastwards on the lowed plains and flat lands of the area around Kilimanjaro. The fast speed of the water did not support aquatic life like fish but the stones and sand were a source of building material at the later years. The stream had its dangers to swimmers. When rain falls in the mountain, the stream filled up and the increased water flow could reach the residential parts without awareness to those in the stream with fatal consequences to anyone in it. The greater water flow carries stone and the noise was a warning sign but that usually was after the fast early silent flow. Youngsters swimming were always told to listen to steam noises of increased water flow, and move to safety promptly. The fast flow destroyed areas known to have natural pools for bathing and swimming and created new ones that had to be discovered. The stream also provided a series of unique plants from the forest. The violent stream carries plants that start growing when deposited as the water speed reduces. The plants were of known medicinal use, good forage for

21

animals or forest climbers that were used as twine in hut building.

The first wife, Mkasu:

Mkasu, Salema's first wife was a small pretty woman, possibly four feet and five inches tall (1.33metres), with a constant laughter whenever she was in conversations. She was, however, serious, intelligent and focused. She never expressed her anger in public and there were no records of anyone knowing that they ever had arguments or quarrels with her husband Salema. Mkasu and Salema had a happy household. The happy household did not mean that rude behaviour escaped punishment. One day when Mkasu observed one of her children asking a stranger for a sugar cane, she tolerated that behaviour until the stranger had gone. She unleashed her wrath to the child by a severe beating using a fine branch of a cypress tree. She explained that the begging gave the impression to the village that she did not feed her children well, a kind of village gossip she did not like to be associated with. She was a hard worker and with Salema by her side they were aspiring for great things. She was progressive as she encouraged and supported her children to go to learn to read and write, an opportunity she did not get. She was kind to both family and neighbours. She would share her food to anyone who came in and found her eating, and in an equal measure share the work if one finds her working. There was a village gossip that Mkasu was a woman who fed you knowing that you would need it as she ensured you worked very hard for the food. Possibly she believed in the saying that there is no free lunch.

The village daily chores:

The sounds of cocks crowing, dogs barking, chickens clucking and occasional the mooing of the cows, were noises enough to make Salema wake up; it would be six in the morning. He dressed fast, with his coat and his tyre shoes, took his machete and the sharpening file, and went out

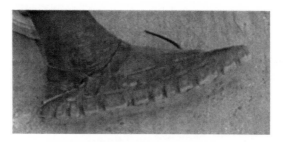

Tyre shoe worn by Salema

happy and cheerful shouting good morning to all his family members to wake up while having a pinch of his snuff. It was another day, his early morning coffee was boiling on the log fire, and the children in every family were getting up to do their morning chores like sweeping inside and around the hut, before going to school. By the time breakfast was ready Salema would have collected enough forage for his in-house kept animals, the kids would

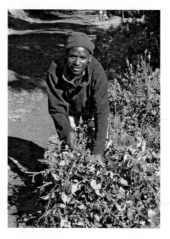

Failosi collecting animal forage

have swept the compound, fetch some forage for their allocated animals then washed, dressed and ready for school. It would then be seven o'clock as classes started at seven thirty prompt, going to school was by running very fast.

When Salema was eating his breakfast he noticed his wife's belly and could not help saying something. All he could say was *'how are you feeling my dear?'* The words fell on deaf ears as Mkasu did not answer, since she assumed he should know. She was in her own deep thoughts that a woman would not tell a man as she believed men would not understand. Her thoughts were not dreams like Salema's but real issue of concern like the expected birth, the pain, the baby's health, the sex or name the celebrations, the presents, and the baby-sitting plans and so on and so on! Mkasu told Salema that the baby was kicking much stronger therefore the days were near. Salema's heart rate increased as he realised an increase of his responsibilities. He left quickly after his breakfast that consisted of tea with milk and sugar, roast unripe bananas and finally a cup of fermented milk. The first place was to weed his corn *'shamba'*—the small plot of land where food and cash crops are cultivated using basic tools like a hoe and machete. The second place to weed was his millet patch. That back breaking job involved kneeling down, and removing the weeds almost one by one with a knife or a pointed stick as the millet seeds are scattered closely so spacing the millet plant is also part of the weeding activity. The millet was a major ingredient in the popular home brew that is known as *'mbege'*.

Weeding that product always filled Salema with the memories of the good times of drinking and enjoyment; including the happiness the product brought to the communities during ceremonies. That time however, weeding brought about the thoughts of the expected child and how much *'mbege'* he would need. His thoughts started to mirror those of his wife. The day was getting too hot to weed under the sun therefore Salema moved to his banana plantation where the cooler temperature enabled him to prune his coffee or space and re-plant some bananas. Working in banana plantation, Salema took the opportunity to check the number of bunches that could be used to make *'mbege'*. As the evening was approaching Salema prepared more forage for his in-house kept animals and headed home to wash, change to clean clothes and go to his friends to socialise to conclude the day. That was a typical normal day for Salema and many of his colleagues in the village of Nanjara. Almost every evening, the drinking *'mbege'* concluded the day.

The social events with the alcoholic beverage called 'mbege':

It is a Chagga peoples' tradition that socializing always included a meeting of people of similar age, usually the elders, at a home of one of the villagers, chat about the weather, usually rains and the crops, drinking of *'mbege'*, and a bit of singing to conclude the day. If there was a child born, the social event could include an additional eating of barbequed lamb meat and more pronounced singing.

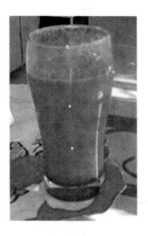

Mbege in a glass

25

'Mbege' was a drink made from ripened bananas, boiled almost to become red, left for a day or two to cool, when water is added during filtration through a bed of reed grass to obtain a cloudy reddish sweet liquid that was left to ferment. That liquid was flavoured by the malt made from the finger millet and the speed of fermentation is regulated by the addition of *'msesewe'*. That was a bitter tasting liquid obtained from boiling the bark of species *'rauwolfia caffra'* The process took seven days to prepare and only good enough to drink for three days as it had storage maximum of three days after which it started to change to vinegar. *'Mbege'* drinking was possible on a daily basis as there was communication among friends to a planned production to cover most of the days of the week. That was the only social activity in the village apart from community work for adults. It was after work that men followed later by their wives, met, chat, exchange ideas, acquire knowledge, and drink *'mbege'*. It was during such gatherings that friendships were made or broken. That was also the most important forum for solving disputes. Any Chagga dispute would not be considered by the elders who were the natural judges; without the availability of *'mbege'*. The community work in the village included communal crop weeding, huts or barns building. In such group work, *'mbege'* was also essential. The older children, who had finished school usually socialise similarly on Sundays after church, where music dancing and drinking took place. The making or breaking of friendships and the possibility of meeting a future wife, were factors that made such gatherings very popular. Younger children of school age had to invent their own social activities. Washing clothes by the river, having a bath in the river, and scrubbing their hard skins off their feet as they did not have shoes to wear and swimming in the river,

use of catapults to prove accuracy of shooting, were the boys' best pastimes. Looking after cattle after school, chopping wood, making wooden carts, wheelbarrows and

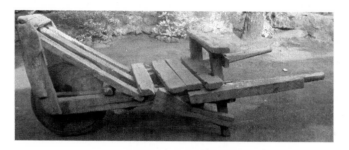

Wooden wheelbarrow

bicycles were other activities that the young boys liked to do. The making of catapults and shooting down birds was an exciting pastime. In a successful hunt boys would start a fire and roast a killed bird. Some birds would not fall to the ground when killed making it essential that boys learned to climb trees to retrieve their hunt. The girls of school age were more homely with their mothers, played hide and seek on their way to collect water or firewood. They accompanied the boys to the river to wash clothes and scrub their feet but never in swimming as the boys swam fully naked.

After a brief wash, Salema left alone, as his wife could not accompany him for obvious reasons, to go to Makinafu for a drink. The topic of conversation was babies. It was not a secret that Mkasu was pregnant, as the whole village knew; therefore they took the liberty of asking Salema many questions and even offered lots of advice. As the drinking at Makinafu's place continued and some people started to feel tipsy, Salema found surrounded by many drinkers each giving advice on the birth of his unborn child and some asking questions, but the most annoying were those predicting the sex of the child. Salema was a quiet well mannered person. He portrayed shyness but he was not a coward. He also took chances in some projects but very careful in his judgement so he avoided hazards. His good character of kindness but not an extravagant person earned him respect. His friend Makinafu detected that he was not happy with the barrage of suggestions, advice and comments; therefore he beckoned him to a private place for a one to one talk. Makinafu, a senior to Salema in age, explained to him the customary issues and Salema listened carefully as he wanted to please especially his father Shenji who was very difficult to please. Makinafu started by reminding Salema the usual story he had to tell his two older siblings. The story as retold was that when the children woke up to find their mother with a baby, they were told that *'when the parents went to the forest to get some logs for the fire, they heard among the bushes a cry and by looking around they found a baby and brought the baby home for the mother to look after:'* The little children would ask to hold and kiss the baby and that was the start of the siblings bond. Salema had to get hold of some logs to show to confirm the story, therefore, Makinafu offered some logs to be collected as the soon as the baby was born. An extra calabash of *'mbege'* made Salema a bit more talkative so he asked some questions like the type of animal to slaughter and when to celebrate the birth and if there was much he could do to please his father. That time Salema wanted to take charge, he did not want his father to do all the rituals as he did for the previous two siblings. Makinafu carefully stirred Salema in the right direction. If it was a boy, a *'horo'* a male goat, was to be slaughtered and must cut the meat traditionally to ensure the new mum gets the best meat and not to forget his father who had to eat the chest *'kidari'* and most important there must be some '*mbege*' available. Makinafu concluded by re assuring Salema that he would keep some brew for emergency. With that friendship note, Salema left heading home through the winding foot paths in the pitch of darkness and singing happily because he was relaxed and that by hearing the singing his wife would have his dinner ready. It was not only his wife who heard the songs but his mother Yohana who confronted him warning him of too much drink when he may expect a child anytime and that he must have his faculties at all times to make the correct preparations. His mother wanted to see him taking the lead in the child's birth ceremony not Shenji who was always very bossy. On various contacts she made this aspiration clear to Salema. Salema was polite to his mother, left without argument, went into the hut to eat his supper and proceeded to his own hut to sleep. His wife always made sure Salema's hut was warm kept that way by a log fire. His mother's words and the fact he must show leadership, made him think again on how to make all he desired possible and not to let his father take charge again. With his mother's words ringing in Salema's head, he barely slept but was in deep thoughts of planning for success. He came to the conclusion that to gain support from wife, mother, and friends, he had to work, even harder than his father.

Salema the tree planting expert:

In his youth, Salema, the second son of Yohana and Shenji, aspired to expand his horizons by going to the city of Nairobi to find a better standard of living. It was in his attempt to get work that he found it difficult as he neither knew how to read nor write. That handicap made him realize that he had to depend on the land for his survival. It was in that struggle of finding work that an English gentleman he met employed him. Salema had to move to Arusha as a hand in assisting the forester. It was during the times of work in the forest care that he learned how to saw seeds, plant tree seedlings, watering and the care of mature trees, but above all that he appreciated the value of trees financially and environmentally on aspects of soil erosion, climate modulation such as rain capture and temperature control. As the years passed he started to think on the task of acquiring a wife. He decided to go home to get a girl from his own village. He could not let down his father by marrying someone from the city and that the activities of city girls did not meet his approval. On his way home, it was the chance meeting with Mkasu that resulted into marriage. When Shenji gave him land, he immediately started planting trees to mark his boundary. The number of trees he planted did not meet hid aspirations so he planted trees in a large part of his land making it look like a forest The only open space was where he turned it into a farm to plant food crops and an area for growing grass for his animals pastures. Salema had a vision that made him consider trees he planted as his *'retirement fund'*. That vision was realised when the sale of the trees as timber funded the education or care of many of Salema's children.

The highly motivated Salema:

Salema made a decision to put his mother' words to practice. He woke up early and started working earlier than anyone even his father. As soon it was possible to see, that is about 5 a.m. Salema would wake up, begin getting forage for his in–house fed animals, (95), and then proceed to the '*shamba*' before breakfast. That new behaviour continued for a good while and was becoming the norm as more and more people noticed and talked about him. The village folk were saying that the hard work was to cover the work of two as his wife could not help. Although that was true, Salema however was aiming to higher ideals that are to take control of all his affairs. It was when his own father commented on his hard work that Salema realised that his efforts were producing dividends, thus boosting his confidence. Fifteen days had passed since Salema was known to be a hard worker and since had achieved respect from his father; he had to keep up the momentum of working hard. The daily routine of working and socializing continued, but some days Salema had to stay home sitting on the thinking stone 'kijiwe'. One day when he had no place to go, Salema resolved to stay at home to relax and think as the evening approached. Salekwa's son came running very fast, as most boys would do when passing information, asking Salema to go to see his father. It was custom that no man sends for another without the prospect of '*mbege*' drinking, so Salema dressed smart, wearing his big coat and walked towards Salekwa's home. Half way on his travel he realised he had forgotten something so he doubled back to see how his wife was before going to meet with his friends. Satisfied that all was well, he went for his drink. At home Mkasu's pain was more frequent but it was not an issue to tell Salema when he came to check on her. The frequencies of contractions become higher, Yohana was called and in turn she called Makakite, the village midwife. The three women, Mkasu, Yohana and Makakite, sat in the hut, keeping the log fire, alive and hot to give extra warmth in the hut. The children,

Salimu and Mkaleso, were sent to the grandfather Shenji, who made sure they never went home until it was safe, in order for the adults to tell convincingly the legendary story of how a baby came to be. Salekwa's brew was not much and each person had only one calabash as it was one of the mid week drinks, so after sunset drinking ended. Dusk and then pitch darkness would follow, making it difficult to go home as Salekwa's place was poorly kept, very bushy and wild. The hard working Salema walked home and as he approached his wife's hut, he noticed a lot of brightness as the kerosene lamps were on and the log fire was optimum. On noticing that change, his heart started racing but he walked slowly towards the door. When he saw Makakite, he asked where Mkasu was, but before he got an answer he saw her in the bed. It was not allowed for a man to be present at birth so he was politely asked to go to bed and wait. Yohana and Makakite had cooked so Salema was given a supper to be consumed at his hut. As he lay on his bed and he started to think, he remembered the wood Makinafu had promised. Despite the late hour, there was some moonlight. That low light enabled Salema to walk to Makinafu to convey the news of possible birth of his third child that night. Preparations to supply the logs at the earliest hour of the morning were made and Salema returned to his hut to wait for news of the birth. He could not sleep therefore he went on thinking, then suddenly he remembered that he had to see his father in case there was something he might have forgotten to do. He put his heavy coat again and walked the short distance to his father's hut for a talk. He was well received, but instead of a long chat his father told him not to panic but to go to sleep. The children were asleep; therefore Salema avoided the question as to why they were at grandpa's place. It was nearly midnight, when he returned to his hut, then he heard some groaning noises from the women's hut but he was not called and he was not allowed entry anyway. He tried to sleep without success; therefore he sat on his folding chair by the log fire gazing into the flames. The soothing effect of the flames induced sleep. It was a moonlit night; the numerous animals were making some slight noises as they perceive it was soon to be daylight. It was not only the noises of animals that woke him up, but also the noises from the women's hut that signified increased activity. He was not called, so he could not go there. The increase of activity made him fully awake and then suddenly he heard a baby cry! He put on his coat to go hoping to be called but the calls never come. The baby's cry continued but that time he also heard some happy chatter among the women, then he heard his name called. As he approached his wife's hut he was told *'it is a boy and all is ok'*. He did not go to see the boy as he was not allowed in; instead he run to his fathers hut to break the news, then to his friend Makinafu.

The birth of Touwa:

Since the cocks had not crowed it was before two o'clock then Salema assumed his son was born at one thirty a.m. on Thursday 15th day of September 1949. He was to be named Touwa, the same name as his wife's father as tradition dictates.

The Chagga tradition has a system of keeping forefathers names in perpetuity by a system of representation into a new family a name from the older generation. That system meant that a first male child represents and may have the name of the husbands father, the second male to represent the wife's father. The girls also followed similarly to represent the mother, then representation of brothers and sisters follow. In Salema's case his second son was then named Touwa, a name after Mkasu's father. Despite that early hour of the morning, Makinafu and Salema enjoyed a calabash of *'mbege'* while discussing the morning's celebration. He did not stay for long as he thought he may be needed anytime for that reason he asked Makinafu to bring the logs early, and to help with some morning chores. With such amicable agreement Salema walked to his hut to rest, as sleeping was not an option.

Salema was so excited, that he had three children, he felt a proper family man who had gained respect that could instantly be lost if he showed failure in their care. He expected well-wishers that day thus he planned to slaughter his fattest male goat ('*horo*')and to obtain some *'mbege'* from neighbours who may have brewed in anticipation of the birth; to add to the amount that he expected would be sent in by friends and family. Satisfied that his plans were in place he got out to check again on his son's few hours' progress. The morning was fast approaching. Salema thought that the whole world was as excited as he was from hearing the sounds of cocks crowing and many of his various animals making their unique calls. That state of being alert made him aware of the mowing cows, bleating goats and sheep, with a chorus of chuckling chickens and quacking ducks, making it clear that there was the wish to be let out to the green pastures. As usual Salema started to get forage for his animals very early; when he was accompanied by Makinafu, and his father Shenji, who helped him with the morning chores but also to gain the scrumptious breakfast prepared by the two women, Yohana and Makakite who performed the midwifery duties. In the morning The breakfast consisted of tea or coffee with roast green bananas, with an additional well seasoned, partially fried then boiled chicken (usually a cockerel)and a cup of fermented milk that brought the birthday breakfast to an end, but signalling the start of a four day long celebration of animal slaughtering, meat eating, *'mbege'* drinking, lots of chatting with singing and dancing.

On Thursday morning, Touwa's first day, Salema slaughtered a goat, friends brought drinks and there was a party till late.

On day two, the same crowd came to check if all was well but also to see if anything was left over, and since there was food, there was a party until late.

On day three, to make it possible to have a good party, two friends, Makinafu and Salekwa, brought meat and *'mbege'* respectively. Shenji, the baby's grandfather, was impressed on seeing his son's success in the ceremonies so he wanted also to make a mark.

On Sunday it was Shenji's day when he offered his son a fat large ram goat to celebrate his grandson's birth. That grandson was special to Shenji, he represented the in-laws; the father of Mkasu, Touwa who was in the ruling family of junior chiefs. The privilege of having this name in his family made Shenji a happy man to celebrate the birth of Touwa his grandson. The news that Shenji was having a drink on the Sunday at his son's place travelled like wild fire and anyone who knew Shenji including the in-laws, Touwa and his friends were expected to be there. After attending church in the morning, Sunday the 17th September Salema registered at the church office the birth and for baptism of his son, before rushing, to go home to prepare for the grand party. There were two areas the visitors would sit, the inner group and the outer rank.

The first grand party for Touwa;

In the inner group, Shenji and Salema's close friends and their wives sat on folding chairs. That group consisted of people who share slaughtered meat and brew regularly including special invited guests like the in laws.

The outer group consisted of any one who wanted a brew, the younger folk with no home of their own yet built and casual friends from other villages. They sat on anything ranging from benches, banana or tree trunks, stools, stones or folding chairs if there were any left.

That separation offered a better social interaction as there was no dissatisfaction as both parties drank the same '*mbege*' fetched from the same barrel. Roast meat was offered to all, and above all that the host, Salema would go round and talk to all. That Sunday there was enough for all. They came thirsty and hungry and they were going home full and satisfied and may have been a bit drunk. The chat turned into singing and eventually dancing. The outer group did not anticipate or believe they would drink and eat that much. To show appreciation, they started singing and by holding hands to make a circle, the singing was so loud such that individuals and eventually the whole of the inner group joined to make the singing even louder and enjoyable. The women also joined. The men and women stood making a ring circle, holding hands, singing and dancing. Dusk was approaching so a log fire was started to give warmth, light, and a focus point for the dancing, as the fire was in the centre of the dancing loop. That was sweet music without instruments. But that was not all. Listening to the lyrics could make a bystander enjoy the party. The songs would start by praising Shenji for his party and for the child, Salema who also got the child that gave them that good food they had eaten. They even praised Touwa for the daughter who had been the reason for the celebration. As the drinking increased, the songs became more comic. The notable one in memory was; '*Oh hauyese, ngalya ngayuta, hauyese ngalya ngalemwa . . . .*' *and* repeating. That was literally translated to '*please go there again as I have eaten, I am full, and can eat no more*' In fact this was a coded message telling Salema to do again what he did to get a baby and that they might get a chance again to enjoy. Songs like those would go on and on with the closest neighbours continuing almost to midnight. At intervals some controversial songs that could criticize a person and praise their enemies were used to air some grievances but that time all good things prevailed.

Life after the birth of Touwa:

Early in the morning Salema woke up as usual accompanied by very early well wishers to carry out his morning chores. Those well wishers came with the expectation of getting good breakfast possibly made from left-over food and an added calabash of brew. In Salema's home they were not disappointed but they worked hard for it. It was a day of mixed work and pleasure where visitors helped to clear the party mess while having a calabash of brew. As many hands are said to make labour light, it was not long before the place was tidy. Drinking started again soon after the arrival of Shenji who came to congratulate his son and to see his grandson. Salema was relaxed and more confident and that time he truly enjoyed by taking part in the singing that followed. That time the brew was finished. Some people would add a little water in the barrel to extract the last drinkable liquid. The next day all the brew barrels were washed and for almost a week Salema's home became for a brief period, 'booze free zone'. It was after all the parties that Salema could think more clearly, had time to kiss and cuddle his second son, Touwa. Touwa as he was called was developing well and Mkasu, his mother, was well rested, well fed, and well cared for. That pampering would continue on a reducing scale for three months, when a small party that involved a slaughter of a sheep to signify the end of pampering. It was after that period that Mkasu would participate fully in the family chores leaving Touwa to a baby sitter, his older sister Mkaleso with the help of grandmother Yohana.

The care of Touwa:

Babysitting was a very hard job for a youngster like Mkaleso who was only four years old. Grandma Yohana was the main baby sitter, encouraging and mentoring Mkaleso. It involved cleaning the baby's bottom using special smooth leaves of the *'ilaka'* bush, which had added beneficial healing properties in the event of a nappy rash. There was also the duty of washing the soiled nappies. In the days of

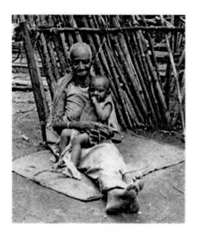

Baby sitting by Yohana

Touwa, nappies were not disposable but towelling type of cotton clothes which had to be washed after every episode of soiling. It was usually a rectangular piece of fabric folded to a triangular shape and tied around the child's bottom with a pin or by a knot. Other baby sitting duties included feeding, watching and talking to the baby and finally ensuring comfort at all times. There was no ready made baby food thus after three months, in addition to breast milk, Touwa was given ripe, boiled or roast bananas made to a fine pulp with mild home made butter, plain milk, fruits and juices. Harder foods that could not be pulped were chewed mostly by the mother or sister and fed from mouth to mouth. That act may look crude but it was a means of supplying nutrient to a baby to a wide variety of adult foods like meat, corn, beans and yams. There were other benefits like partially digesting the food for the baby. That was how Touwa was fed.

Village life confidential:

Life in the village including Salema's household was back to normal as the excitement of child birth, celebrations, drinking, eating and singing were over. Normal life in the village involved the early waking up to get animal feed, letting the free range animals to the green pastures, cultivating, planting, weeding or harvesting, depending on the season. Men and boys usually were cattle herders, coffee tenders, and planted and propagated banana plants including cultivation and harvesting the seasonal crops. Women and girls cultivated the food plots too, fetched wood and water, milked the cows, and cooked. In some families boys were made to milk cows or to fetch water signifying that division of labour was not strict.

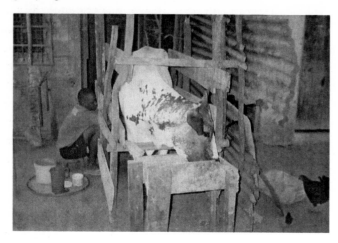

Cow milking

Most evenings, the men made an attempt of being nice by chopping the large logs, for fire, then say they are tired as an excuse to escape to go for a drink of *'mbege'*. To be nicer, on their way home, the men usually brought back a calabash of *'mbege'* to their wives. In the night, one can hear men singing loudly on their way home, may be because they were very happy, but also, because every one sang rather loudly there was a reason. It came to be known that, in the land where many a man had more than one wife, the singing was to alert the wife to get food ready but also to warn admires in the event they may be visiting, to get out! Stories had emerged that many confrontations were thus avoided despite known cases of children that resembled the quiet village fellow rather than the man they called father! Most women knew signs to look for to detect infidelity but not a single word was uttered in public. The children like Touwa grew up in happy friendly village unaware that adults had some secrets. The big secret was that the old man Shenji was known to have amorous tendencies towards a number of the village women and with the possibility of fathering children. Yohana, his wife had three children, Mkosi, Salema and her third child, a girl, called Rosalia. It was after the birth of that younger sister of Salema that Shenji embarked on a marriage to a second wife Mamacholo. Shenji and Mamacholo had four children. Their names were Sumaili, Kimwai, Failosi and Benadina. Yohana, Shenji's first wife was rebellious and was the first tension between Shenji and Yohana that led to life changing events that made growing up in the green pastures of home memorable and educational but above all determined the future and the path that the family followed. That rebellion by Yohana took a practical dimension when she moved and lived with his son after he was married. Yohana moved from Shenji's hut to live with his son's family and take the duties of baby sitter. Salema gained a pair of hands to ease the daily chores, and Mkasu gained a baby sitter.

Yohana, Touwa's beloved grandmother:

In addition to all these benefits that she brought to his son's family after abandoning Shenji, Yohana had a good knowledge of herbs to cure many ailments. Notable was the use of leaves of a bush known as *'mshang'a'*, an excellent cure for tape worms, a worm infestation that was common to many of the village children. Chewing and swallowing these leaves or drinking the juices, helped Touwa to avoid the stigma of having tape worms in his growing up years. When tape worms infect a person, the segmented worms would grow symbiotically inside the persons gut sharing the nutrients. For growing children that infestation was detrimental to health. When one had tape worms, it was a sign of being dirty and was kept as a secret. But that was one infection that could not be kept secret. As the worms grew in the gut, segments detached, slid down through ones back passage without their realisation and fell on the calf muscles of the legs. Anyone walking behind the person could see the infestation, a white flat segment of a worm. It was a mark of great shame to be known to have tapeworms and teasing was common among all age groups.

The duties of babysitting that Yohana undertook, enabled her to progress in her excellent story telling qualities that he portrayed to her grandchildren irrespective of age. The stories were based on forest animals and the danger they posed on humans especially children. The most frightening of her stories was about a little girl who went to visit her grandmother away across the forest to find that the grandmother had big ears, big teeth and long sharp nails. The grandchildren slept in grandmother's hut because they were very frightened. The curiosity of the children to know how stories ended was that powerful as they requested grandma to continue the story telling the next day after dinner. That quality time of grandma's stories was remembered by all as they grew up.

Story telling was good but Yohana hag also an excellent knowledge in making snuff. The snuff was snorted through the nose or placed between the front lower teeth and the lip. The dark brown powder was meticulously made from tender tobacco leaves dries in the shed flavoured by adding powder from a limestone rock and ground to a fine powder between smooth stones. To enhance smoothness a little nut oil was added during the fine grinding stage. The fine snuff was stored in sachets made by dried banana stem-peel or small containers such as a photo film cover or a tin that was emptied of shoe polish. The snuff was used socially as request for snuff could be a start of conversation, an excuse to be introduced, or even a start of friendship and in some cases it was used as a chat up motivator. Snuff was popular in the days Touwa grew up as he noted that his father, grandma, grandad and all their friends were users. Mkasu was not a user. The grandchildren grew to love their grandmother, with the memories of her stories, her medicines and above all the visitors that came to ask for snuff. That love portrayed a very happy Salema family. That perfect arrangement for Salema family did not escape the wrath of Shenji, who waited for the moment to strike a blow to Yohana, his wife and Salema, his son for deserting him by showing boldness in his independence to his father as he regained his confidence, a state interpreted by his father as desertion, may be with a little jealousy.

Family cohesion tested:

Shenji was starting to indicate his displeasure but had to cool down as there was little he could do immediately when Touwa became ill. Tensions were put aside as the little boy on his first birthday was afflicted with a serious illness. Touwa caught whooping cough, a fatal childhood disease that took away the lives of many children in the village. Mkasu took Touwa to the small dispensary, manned by a Medical Assistant who was trained to perform the duties of a Doctor, as he diagnosed, a Nurse, as he bandaged wounds, as a Pharmacist as he dispensed medicines; and a Surgeon, as he performed minor surgeries like circumcisions.

That broadly trained man did all he could to alleviate suffering due to ill health in the community and it was all done well. Touwa was given the medication available and sent home to recover. Whooping cough was a cruel disease for a child, who would cough constantly with the sticky, elastic mucus that was pushed out on the cough reflex to be inhaled again on the breathing in reflex, filling the lungs, nostrils and mouth with the tendency to choke and suffocate. Mkasu and Salema nearly believed that their child would die. Salema could only write his name nothing else, so he took a piece of charcoal and a paper from the elder brothers writing book, put Touwa's foot on the paper and traced the shape of the sick little boy's foot and kept it in his memory in the event that he died. Mkasu, Touwa's mum did all he could to keep the boy alive, giving of medicine sometimes via mouth to mouth delivery. She took to herself as the most personal act of love; use her mouth to suck the mucus from the nose and mouth of her child to give him the ability to breath. Each passing day was touch and go; the worry over the little boy was constant over a two month's period before few signs of recovery were observed. The family union was at its peak during the sad times. Yohana observed that Touwa slept better ate a little more and showed signs of the need to move and play. At one year and two months Touwa was over the worst, the parents were looking forward to his recovery, which was manifested by walking and talking more and more. Life in the family returned to normal, and even Shenji was in a reconciliatory mood, as a result peace was regained. Salema continued to work hard, his bumper crop that year was another boost to his confidence and after selling the crops he had cash to spare and he felt rich. He wisely spent his excess cash by building the then first house of the family Unlike the hut the new house was a two room house—a sitting room and a bedroom. The walls were

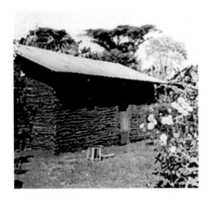

made of a wood structure, plastered with mud. It had windows and two doors front and back with the roof thatched with corrugated aluminium sheets. It was a grandeur design, showing progress in the village. It was very noisy when the tropical rains fell but very soothing during

Salemas modern house

periods of light rains but admired by all in the village and many people copied that design. Salema's father, Shenji, approved that new house design as it signified progress. Salema used that new house as his bedroom sharing it with his sons without animals, pets or log fires. His ego did not end with that new house, he went on to build a bigger and better store like a silo for his food products, beans, maize and the

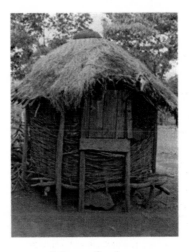

Salemas food store

finger millet which was used for making *'mbege'*. His confidence did not stop there. Salema built a bigger barn to accommodate the increasing number of animals that kept on growing from additions of cattle and sheep given to Touwa by his grandfather who intended to give him a hold on the property ladder. Touwa was growing healthier, as he could walk a distance from the huts in order to play with other youngsters. Village life was now normal again with children laughing and playing. Adults were heard chatting and gossiping happily, girls going to fetch water giggling louder, women calling their siblings to eat their food and the men sniffing for the pleasant smell of *'mbege'* brew after their work in the *'shamba'* to determine who had some the local brew ready to drink.

Old habits die hard:

Those evenings of social life had some serious drawbacks as it was during those periods of intoxication that temptations start to surface as the opposite sex seemed to look prettier or more handsome in proportion to the amount of *'mbege'* drank. Salema was not immune to those temptations. After his third child was born, just like his father before, Salema made the old mistake of marrying a second wife. Mkasu was furious! The new woman felt unwelcome but she did not leave, resulting in tensions that got so heated, that Salema who was in the middle, could not take any more pressure. Salema could neither throw her out nor keep her in a hut near his first wife, as there was the possibility of a pregnancy.

Shenji intervened, to solve the family crisis by suggesting a piece of land for Salema to build a hut for the new wife.

Yohana, Salema's mother had experienced such an incident and reassured Mkasu to cool down as there was little that could be done citing her personal experience. Yohana wanted to keep her new family intact and functioning as good as possible. It was during reconciliatory talks between Yohana and Mkasu that a serious decision that influenced the future of the family was made.

Mkasu asked Yohana to care for her children with the help of her younger sister Atanasia, who was married and living a short distance from her. She stressed that Yohana should never allow Salema to involve the new wife in any caretaking of her children, whether she was alive or dead. The fragile truce existed but from then on Salema was not so happy again. Salema had to find a way out especially after the birth of Ndesumbuka, Touwa's younger brother. At that time Touwa was two years old. The fragile peace was destroyed when the new wife gave birth to a girl, Kibasi. That birth caused so much tension that Salema could not bear the strain; he opted to leave home, away from his two wives to find some calmness somewhere.

He found a plot of land almost forty hectares, of virgin bush on the boundary between Kenya and Tanzania. He made a temporary shack and worked the land which was very fertile. The harvest from that land was very high. It increased Salema's cash flow. With gained confidence he returned to his two wives ensuring they had enough money to look after the children. Despite that good gesture, Salema found out those tensions still simmered. He had little choice but to go and live in solitude in the new farm or as it was known, the Boundary Farm. That good gesture of Salema toward his wives was to ensure no suffering occurred as a result of his actions. Time is said to heal, because it was observed that Salema's effort in the provision of supplies, food, money, and his absence reduced the fury of the women towards him as he was acting as a 'good' husband. Life was returning to near normal but Salema chose to stay at the boundary farm in solitude.

The second wife—Alina:

Alina, the second wife of Salema was a shy lady, not very talkative but when confronted, she knew how to defend herself. She must have loved Salema very much or Salema must have impressed her that much that she agreed to be a second wife. Although it was generally accepted for a man to marry more than one wife, a woman who became involved in a polygamous relationship encountered lots of abuse, hatred and animosity in the early years prior to establishing herself in the complex family set up. Alina was kind to Mkasu's children as Mkasu, the first wife showed no hatred to the children of Alina As the year progressed Alina worked hard and was able to have her own land and home for her children. The children of Alina and those of Mkasu grew in a friendly family atmosphere as the parents problems were not aired in public to involve the children, making Salema's family a complex one but united.

Life of Solitude in the boundary farm:

It was not known exactly how Salema gained the confidence of his two wives, but one thing was true; that there was normality in their relationships, because his wives were having more children. The harvest from the new farm made him better off financially and the motivation to continue despite his fragile domestic arrangement. In his new farm Salema encountered crop damage by wild animals through eating or just passing through, a pattern mostly carried out by elephants. Salema was full of ideas and one of those thoughts could be a solution to his crop damage problem. He pleaded with his friends to join him to open farms near the boundary farm as he realised that more farms would drive the wild animals away to the forest or the new farms if with crops would act as a buffer to protect his own farm or the animals would have enough to eat without emptying the farms. His call to join him in the boundary farm fell on deaf ears but one man was not amused. Shenji thought that his son Salema was driving people away from the village he established, the people he encouraged to join him and he felt betrayed by his own son and opened the old wounds, the issues that prior to Touwa's illness.

That was the basis of disapproval by Shenji that was simmering slowly with the potential of a dispute. When no one listened to Salema to join him, Shenji was happy that his son failed in that plan. He thought Salema was becoming too big for his boots and that he was forgetting all his father had done for him that is, giving him his first piece of land. Despite that failure Salema pressed on developing his boundary farm, the year that followed his harvest was large, and he was noticeably wealthy. He built a shop to buy grain from the villagers for sale to the big towns. The shop was successful for the first year but things turned sour when some relatives offered to take the grain to town to sell but kept the money and promised: *'I will bring the money to tomorrow'*, but then 'tomorrow' never came. Salema was not educated but he was wise and clever enough to see that it was not the way business was conducted, so he shut the shop. Many in the village noticed Salema's wealth and embarked on joining him to develop areas around the boundary farm. They built shacks and huts, and with a short time the boundary farm area became a village.

Salema was now a leader, (pictured with family and friends enjoying a drink after work) even his wives joined

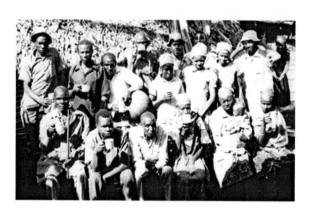

Salema and family at boundary farm

him to help in the farm but in the evening the wives had to leave. He preferred his peace therefore no one was invited to stay. He, however, visited his wives and was a member of the Nanjara village again. With the passing years, Salema fathered more children. Before the start of the boundary farm Salimu, Mkaleso, Touwa and Ndesumbuka were born. During the development of the farm Melikoi, Tabuni and Tabu were born and Mkasu had seven children—one girl and six boys. Alina, the second wife had Kibasi, Yonaa, Serbi, Mshiki and Vangindele a total of six children, three boys and three girls.

The birth of each child caused serious tensions in Salema household and it was Shenji who played a pivotal role to hold the family in a peaceful state. Shenji performed all the ceremonies for each child born irrespective of the mother as both wives were having the children almost simultaneously. He gave each new born child a goat, a sheep and a cow to help them up the property ladder. Feeding these animals required hard work that kept the mothers very busy, as the harder a woman worked, the more respect she gained from the men, other women and family. Shenji was keeping the women busy to let his son get some peace. In fact Shenji had mixed feelings for his son, paramount was love for the hard work he did, but also there was disapproval for leaving the Nanjara village to go to live in the boundary farm. Shenji, his father felt lonely but despite all these differences, the family happiness was paramount to Shenji.

Growing up in the green pastures:

Shenji's love for his grandchildren united the family, made the women respect or tolerate one another without bickering. The children played together and above all the children were allowed to eat at any of the wives' homes. As the years passed, Touwa was growing up well, was healthy clever and always in a happy mood. At the age of four Touwa knew the whole village as he could pass messages to the elders, or go to buy sugar, salt or matches from the shop for his mother. He also learned how to earn money. He noted that his elder bother and sister collect the grain that has fallen to the ground during harvest. The grain so collected was taken to the shop to sell; the money was immediately used to buy sweets. It was during one of his visits to the shop to sell his grain that Touwa heard some rude jokes. Touwa was called to a group of older boys gathering around the shop. One boy told Touwa to ask his sister to go to him to collect the ripe banana because it was ready. Without any understanding what it meant Touwa went home did not see his sister so he told his mother! In a sudden act of fury his mother gave Touwa a severe beating with a whip. He never repeated those words again and he never knew what they meant until when he was much older.

During his trips to the shop, Touwa noted that the school children had new clean clothes and would not play with him as he was dirty. He thought that if he went to school he would be clean and get new clothes. That was his main motive for going to school. Touwa started following his older brother to half way towards school, but later he got braver and followed him to the school. His big brother noticed him before he could return home. Touwa had not gone so far from home before that it was possible he could be lost if he returned home alone, for that reason Salimu took him to the '*kindergarten*' class where he could stay to wait for him so that they could go home together. When the teacher agreed, it was the happiest moment for Touwa, as he saw a school and inside a class for the first time. He did not know what to do so he sat like the other children; he behaved well, he was keen to learn and impressed the teacher. At noon when his brother collected him to go home, the teacher told him to ask his father to bring him for registration.

Registration to start school was easy. A teacher holds a child's right hand, move it above the head to touch the left ear. When the finger touches the ear, one was old enough that is aged six or over to start school. Touwa was in line almost the last as he was very small but also he could be the youngest, he was not yet six. When it came to Touwa's time to check, the teacher remembered him and without checking he said OK. Touwa ran fast into the classroom to tell the registering staff his name. Salema was delighted, he promised him new clothes and when he reached home, Mkasu, his mother promised him new church clothes. That was the start of school and the road to studying for Touwa.

Life of a school kid:

On his first day at school, the teacher checked, if hair was cut and combed, hands, nails, face and behind the ears washed, clothes cleaned and ironed That first lesson in hygiene was followed by a cleaning task to keep the school compound tidy with the added duty to pick up discarded papers or other articles.

The class started by reciting a,b,c . . . and 1,2,3, ... followed in later days to writing on small framed slates using slate pencils. The slates were delicate such that too much pressure on the slate when writing could break the slate but too weak writing did not scratch the board sufficient to be seen. In '*kindergarten*' it took time to find the balance. Touwa achieved the art of writing on a slate using his left hand but he was unable to use his right hand even after actions from some teachers that included punishments. He was eventually allowed to use his left hand when the Head teacher was making inspection and noted his good writing with the left hand compared with the use of the right hand. That freedom to use the left hand in writing was the start of Touwa's improvement to catch up with his new friends Shirima and Failosi.

Life at '*kindergarten*' was good as it mainly involved making of friends who in turn had a nick name for Touwa. The new friends called him '*Kachwi*' the smallest bird, as he was small and petite. He loved that nick name. His popularity increased as well as his reading and writing, with an added bonus of being promoted to Standard one. The year one in lower primary school was the start of a period of four years measured by standards from one to four. One had to pass an annual examination in order to get a higher standard. Failure meant repeating the same class or even demoted to a lower class, therefore working hard was of essence.

In standard one, there was more in writing, reading more books and introduction to arithmetic, which was, addition and subtraction of numbers. There were more things to learn like school songs and also gardening, a lesson that pleased Touwa's father, Salema as he wanted his children to excel in better farming methods. In his youth Salema worked in a forestry setting where he learnt how to plant and care for trees. He applied his knowledge by planting trees all around his farms both at Nanjara and at the boundary. Touwa was growing well and thought he could join his father at the boundary farm, an idea that was rejected by his mother on fear of being eaten by wild beasts as this farm was a wild forest.

When Touwa passed his examinations and was promoted to a higher class there was happiness at the family home. That was a great change as the school day was then the whole day, requiring the need for a packed lunch. Each pupil needed something to eat in the middle of the day and their mothers prepared packed lunches. Food for lunch consisted of a small choice of staple dishes that were made in the village. The food was wrapped carefully in such a manner that some dishes were still warm at lunch time. A clean soft, young banana leaf was carefully warmed over a wood fire. That process made the leaf soft and flexible with a feel like plastic sheet or grease proof paper. The processed leaf was used to wrap food, two layers kept the food warm by lunchtime. Two or three dry banana leaves were used as outer covering. The resulting food parcel attained a shape of an earthen cooking pot. That was Touwa's lunch box. The unique method of wrapping food was used by travelling people when they travelled great distances to exploit virgin lands as was done by Shenji, Touwa's granddad. The three friends, Touwa, Shirima and Failosi always share their lunch because they were also neighbours. No one ate lunch alone, there was always sharing, an act that helped to build a community spirit and cement some friendships. Some people would bring boiled corn or corn with beans, bananas with or without meat and the most popular dish, corn meal usually known a 'ugali' That mix was of boiled water and maize flour, attained a stiff texture after vigorous stirring while heating with the final cooked product that looks like cake. '*Ugali*' was never eaten without relish. It is the relish that makes it good or poor food. Good '*ugali*' was when the relish was meat, beans, greens, or mild sour milk. Roast or boiled bananas with meat was another popular dish. The foods judged as good were used to make friends, as an invitation to eat together was a sign of respect and friendship. If one

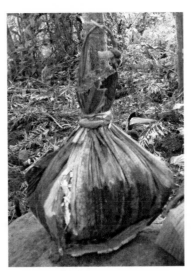

Lunch box in school days

made an invite, one was also invited. The social interaction at lunch times shaped the social life of many lower primary school pupils. Good lunch box was therefore a mark of respect, status and family dignity. Friendships broke when some individual could eat a friend's good food just to give poor quality food. It was an accepted fact that it was better to ask or beg for dinner than to offer bad food.

Life in standard two was filled with surprising new subjects like Geography, History, reading and story telling. Notable of the stories was that of Kalumekenge who refused to go to school. That story was well rehearsed and pupils knew it so well they went home to tell their younger brothers or sister and to their parents. There was a rumour that pupils who learned that story went on to tell their children and grandchildren. That story was loved as it followed chain events using a series of characters well known locally namely, a whip, fire, water, a cow, and a butcher. Those set of characters first refused to help then eventually they were persuaded by a slight threat, to force Kalumekenge, who eventually went to school.

School gardening was a learning process, unlike village farm work. In school, a more programmed type of gardening was done. The pupils planted new food products, like cabbages, carrots, lettuce, onions in straight lines, and properly spaced including how to water and prevent parasites.

Sports activities like football were well organised, in contrast to children playing. These new and organised school activities made going to school a good thing for many children as they were partially exempted from the back breaking work of fetching fodder for animals or working in the farm. Some children however, thought that if they leave home and pretending to go to school but not attending school, that would be avoiding both types of work. Failosi with other kids tried that plan and found it worked. Touwa joined the truancy group to check whether it was fun. Playing and not doing anything while eating cane sugar was fun. That fun made Touwa an absentee from school for a week. A chance meeting of Mkasu, by Shirima, his friend, who asked if Touwa was alright as he had not been seen in school for a week. Mkasu replied that he was a bit unwell but he would be in school the following week. She realised Touwa's trick on truancy. She got a long flexible branch of a cypress tree for use as a whip then went home in a livid mood. At the time school closed Touwa arrived home as usual. His mother gave him food, as usual, but that time a question was asked about the state of his uniform's cleanliness. From his mother's voice which was slightly raised, Touwa knew the game was over. He cried profusely, knelt at his mother's feet, told the whole truth, and even who was involved. Mkasu could not beat Touwa as she had planned, because the truth was revealed in heart felt sincerity and that the boy would not attempt truancy again. That time he was spared a serious beating. He promptly went to wash his clothes on that weekend, ironed, cleaned himself well and was ready for school the following Monday. When his father heard about the truancy, he was furious; he did not hesitate to take Touwa to the boundary farm where truancy would mean being eaten by wild animals. That time Mkasu allowed Touwa go to the boundary farm to face a tougher existence. Shenji, the grandfather, also heard about the truancy, he started to shout loudly calling Touwa to go and see him. That was a terrifying moment for that little boy who made Shenji angry. Everyone in the village was afraid of making Shenji angry, so Touwa approached Shenji's hut with his pants already wet. The granddad stopped shouting as Touwa entered the hut and sat down. With a gentle kind voice, Shenji asked Touwa what he really wanted to do, if given the choice of looking after the animals or going to school. Without hesitation Touwa answered, *'school granddad'*. Shenji expressed happiness and hugged Touwa saying that he could not read or write but he believed that if he was given that education, he would have done better things than he was doing then, and asked Touwa never to be like him but to aspire for bigger and better things that education would offer. From that moment there was a bond, respect and love that blossomed over the years between grandfather and grandson. Touwa re-started school while Failosi's truancy continued and eventually he was out of school. Shirima helped Touwa to catch up with lessons and homework he had missed. Touwa and Shirima were on the path to standard three.

In the new class, in addition to the demand of a higher level of hygiene and cleanliness, gardening and sports, new subjects were introduced like Geography, History and new languages, Swahili and English. In arithmetic there were more new lessons like introduction to division, addition, subtraction and multiplication of larger numbers higher than the times tables. Reasoning in arithmetic was another new subject. Profit and loss calculations were lessons that Touwa's grasp was very poor. Touwa knew that without understanding that lesson he was sure to fail, but for the effort of his friend Shirima who navigated him to an understanding that he then got the questions right. That bond of the two friends was never to be broken.

An incident during play proved that the two friends were formidable. Touwa's short pants had a hole caused by excessive sliding on the river stones making it possible to see his buttocks. His older brother Salimu who took up training as a tailor made the repairs but missed some areas which were like small pockets. Some boys put stones in those little pocket-like spaces. When Touwa entered the class and sat down, he cried loudly with pain as he sat on the stones. The matter could have ended there but the group of boys who did that laughed loudly at Touwa. Touwa was furious but just as he wanted to throw the stones in their direction the teacher entered, silence resumed and all stood up to say *'good morning sir'.*

At lunch time Touwa and Shirima planned to beat the boys after school. They deliberated that they were only two boys against five. Hand to hand combat was ruled out. They planned to use *'ndulele'*;a yellow coloured berry that looked like small tomatoes but very firm when squeezed with a pungent smell and very bitter taste when split. When thrown as a missile to someone it caused pain but no cuts. If it smashed on someone's head the smell was more disturbing than the pain. Secretly Shirima and Touwa collected lots of the berries that were in abundance

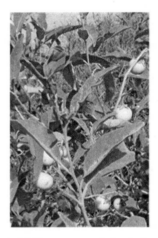

'Ndulele' **berries used for fighting**

along the roadside, to fill all their pockets. The enemy was the group of boys and girls whose homes were across the river Tarakea that mocked Touwa's torn short pants. They were the *'river group'.* The *'forest boys'* consisted of two boys only, namely Shirima and Touwa who lived close to the forest. The last bell for the day was sounded, when all books, pencils, pens and inks were hurriedly gathered and put in the receptacle under the desk when the forest boys run towards home so fast that one could think their homes were also running away. Touwa and Shirima were not running to go home but to lay in wait to ambush with '*ndulele*' fight those naughty and rude '*river group*' boys When the river group boys arrived at the cross road on their way home they were pelted with 'ndulele'. Lots of 'ndulele' broke on the foreheads of many of the boys who did not get a chance of collecting their own missiles. Some girls also were hurt in the cross fire. Many of the boys run home crying while Shirima and Touwa ran towards home now laughing and victorious against the boys who made fun of Touwa's hole on the buttocks area of his pants. The next day, the winning team knew that revenge was in the air, such they enlisted more troops. Their first recruits were Ndesumbuka and Mwandafu, the younger bothers of Touwa and Shirima respectively. The story of the fight was leaked in the class, and it was clear that no one was safe alone, so each person had to identify with a group. The winning team was gaining members but the river group was still much bigger and really furious. It was certain a great fight would ensue that evening after school. At the first dong of the last bell, Touwa and Shirima were almost outside ready with missiles of '*ndulele*'. As the river group got out, they were met with a barrage of '*ndulele*' and had no choice but to run fast homewards. The missiles followed them to the river bank. Hiding in the dry bed of the river, the river group in desperation started using stones for missiles. On detecting that non compliance to the rules of the fight, Touwa, Shirima, and their brothers left and went home without a word leaving the river boys throwing stones for a good while without any opposition.

The story of that fight reached the ears of the Head teacher and the Priest. On Sunday after mass, the Priest called all the school boys and girls and discussed the danger of throwing stones. When the Priest hinted that the Head teacher also knew about the stone throwing, the children were petrified on what was in store for them that following Monday. The *'ndulele'* fight that turned into stone throwing was condemned by the priest, the parents and the Head teacher and so a punishment was certain but one question in the minds of all seniors was who was to be punished. There were names mentioned but there was no definite proof. The Head teacher supported by parents and the priest decided to punish the whole class of standard three.

There was a project in progress to build a classroom or two in order for the school to take more pupils. That project needed the pupils to collect stones and sand from river Tarakea, a kilometre away from the school. The wisdom was Standard three to devote the whole of Monday collecting stones and carrying them from the river to the school. On Monday morning, the standard three was called to meet the Head teacher; the pupils expected a serious physical punishment which was the norm. The head teacher started talking to the trembling class He took a long time, and some pupils started wetting their pants. The punishment was that the forty pupils in standard three would go to the river to collect stones small and large, carry the stones to the school to fill a box that was about a cubic metre. The angry Head teacher then said *'go'*. All the pupils turned and started running towards the river. Each pupil carried as much as they could in order to make the required volume. The smaller and younger boys like Touwa and Shirima and also the girls found it was a really difficult work. The stronger older children found it was a challenge but also fun work. Work continued for the whole of Monday, when the older kids filled the box but the girls and the younger smaller children continued their punishment on the next day and the next until there was a full box of stones. Those who finished early did gardening or sports. The children were very tired; as a result, they never wanted to touch a stone again. Normal classes resumed when the Head teacher accepted that the punishment was done. That punishment had some benefit as it was realised that the total requirement of stones and sand could be collected by the pupils voluntarily one day per week. That policy was implemented and the classrooms were built. It was during those sessions of stone collection that the forest boys made peace with the river boys and there was a good level of bilateral friendships forming including bonding with girls and boys that continued to later years. It was also during those stone collecting sessions that an accident occurred when Touwa was injured. When the pupils were collecting stones and carrying them to the school, they usually threw the stones to the stone pile that was growing. It was during that stone throwing to the pile that a tired girl hit Touwa's left eye with a stone as she threw without looking. It was an accident because it was Touwa's friend, Rita. Rita cried and panicked calling the teacher for help. Touwa was taken to the local dispensary, examined and discharged as there was no blood visible. Touwa's mother nursed her son's swollen eye for a few days and he was well enough to go to school after four days. Shenji was furious as he learned that his son Salema was absent all the time that Touwa was ill. He sent a message calling Salema, and when he arrived a huge family feud erupted.

The conflict:

Shenji had issues that needed resolving, which were his sons disrespect, the issue of Yohana (Salema's mother) staying away from Shenji's hut and the issue of going away far from the village qualified with a hint of jealousy as his son was richer and more influential. Salema also had issues with his father as being too dominant and that Salema felt that as an adult he should not receive anymore orders from his father.

It was late in the night when Yohana, Mkasu and all the children were in their beds when a loud noise of people with machetes cutting banana plants in anger woke up the family. On realising it was Shenji quarrelling with his son, Mkasu grabbed the children, the older children carrying the younger ones and hurriedly running out of the hut to hide in the banana bushes. Mkasu was visibly shaking, as she held Touwa close to her while hiding. Yohana Shenji's first wife stayed put in the hut to confront him as he threatened burning all Salema's huts and throw him out of the land. To save the life of his mother as he knew Shenji's temper did not have limits, Salema started a reconciliatory tone of negotiation in agreement to his father's demands. Shenji realised that if he burned the hut that would kill Yohana and his reputation that was massive would be lost. The exchange of grievances went on between Yohana, Shenji and Salema until cock crowing started. Every one was tired, and Shenji slowly went to his hut and the family went back in the hut but still worried, as periodically Shenji would shout loudly requiring the problem to be settled the following day. Shenji called all the village elders, namely Makinafu, Somboko, Mkosi, Makibonya, Kiberenge, Makimaina, Salekwa, Kitashinja, Mjeuri, Anyika, Yosia, Fidelisi, Manari,

Losina, Shirima, Mausa, Makakite, Mdoko, Kimosoyo and Eskeli the next day to air his disapproval of what his son was doing. A day was set for deliberations when *'mbege'* would have been prepared. It was amazing to see the power that a sitting involving *'mbege'* drinking and meat eating had in finding peace among feuding parties. Makinafu acted as Salema's speaker but Shenji represented himself. It was this arrangement that brought peace as Salema had no direct talk with his father; a strategy that helped to cool down tempers. Makinafu, a long time friend of Salema asked Salema to slaughter the fattest ram. Before it was slaughtered, Makinafu called Shenji to approve it as adequate. When Shenji approved it was almost an open and shut case as Makinafu visualised the strategy for peace. The day came and all the elders assembled. Drinks were in abundance, followed by roast meat. Makinafu did not start until he noted that many elders were relaxed and satisfied with the welcome. When Shenji presented his case all listened in silence as no one was allowed to interrupt him. Makinafu was allowed to reply on behalf of Salema. He started praising Shenji for being the vanguard that brought all the people to the village and gave them land and carefully adding that his son was following his father's footsteps. When the crowd approved, Makinafu felt more confident and told Shenji that what he needed was for his son to say he loved him, as going to a far place is not lack of love, and referred to the quality of the ram slaughtered, Shenji became more approachable, and the seeds of peace were sawn. The party ended with praising songs like : *'haya oh haya haya heee'* which was a chorus after a description of a happy event with dancing that included jumping and stamping feet with the energy of people that signified happiness.

The family routine was back to normal, kids going to school, Salema going to the boundary farm, cattle taken for pastures in the forest, harvesting crops and storage, taking crops to the market and the socializing with '*mbege*' drinking. Touwa was then in the process of writing examinations for completing standard three and he passed to go to Standards four.

The last year in lower primary school was standard four. To go to upper primary school, it was necessary to pass the examinations and gain selection into the limited spaces available. Failure meant that one would be assigned to the village way of life, which meant back breaking farm work. As one grew older, married would be the next step then children or even more wives. Finally with time older age would creep in to find oneself a village elder. The pupils in the Upper Primary school wore very clean white shirts, nice khaki shorts and shoes. Touwa at age eight had never owned a pair of shoes. He therefore thought that to get shoes, it was essential to pass and be selected to go to upper primary school, that was standard five and above. That was his set ambition and he knew how to achieve it by reading and studying in order to learn all he was taught.

When Touwa was nine:

For three days in the week Touwa was living with his dad in the boundary farm. One Thursday morning Touwa woke up to go to school as usual but that morning he did not see his dad to say bye, because he thought his dad had gone to the fields early in the morning, therefore he left and travelled to school. He arrived at school a little early and went past the school to his auntie Atanasia, who lived near

65

the school, to get something to eat as she was a very kind auntie who had always some food to eat. Before Touwa arrived at his auntie, he met Mkaleso, his sister who said nothing but asked Touwa if they could go home. Touwa did not know why and did not question his sister but he just followed to go to the Nanjara home. On the way home they met with their cousin who was going to school. The cousin did not waste time but said to Touwa; *'utaseke namu tewete mayoo'* translated as ***'do not laugh as you no longer have a mother'***. That awfully rude way of breaking bad news was instantly understood by Touwa who ran towards home crying profusely, followed and being comforted by his sister who then started crying profusely. On arrival grandmother Yohana heard them coming, crying, received them, and took them quickly into the hut. Young children were shielded from seeing anything to do with death like the body, digging of the grave or the burial, only to be let out to see the fully covered grave, when they could be encouraged to place some flowers on top. Mkasu, Touwa's mother died aged 36, from complications of child birth on a Wednesday night the month of May 1959, leaving seven children Salimu aged 15, Mkaleso aged 13, Touwa aged 9 Ndesumbuka aged 7 Melikoi aged 5 Tabu aged 2, and Tabuni a baby aged just 13 months. She was laid to rest in a grave,

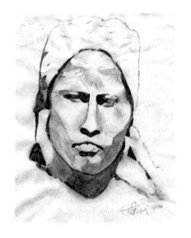

Mkasu artist impression

a few metres from her hut. In his first encounter with death Touwa just made sense of why his father was not at the boundary farm but the consequences of that death were not fully realised. Touwa was constantly observing changes that did not make any sense to him but he was affected. His aunt, Atanasia, a younger sister to the late Mkasu, worked very hard to ensure that all had food to eat and slept well. With Yohana as the rock of the family, the big son Salimu and the only daughter Mkaleso, affairs of the family were handled almost back to normal. There was no part to play by the second wife as it was instructed by Mkasu before her death. Salema kept his grief private lest his children see him crying. He stayed with the children for long hours, during the two weeks of mourning, without much talk but observing each person and planning what to do. First step was that he took Touwa and Ndesumbuka to stay with him at the boundary farm, for few days per week, leaving the baby Tabuni and the other two boys Melikoi and Tabu to live with Grandma Yohana. That was an arrangement that worked according to the wishes of his late wife, Mkasu. A little sign of happiness was a welcome blessing to the family when Touwa was able to continue with his lessons of standard four, and with friends like Shirima, life at home and school was near normal.

School and Exams:

That new class was a great relief for some and seriously a nervous period for others. Those who thought it was a relief, were tired of school and wished for the finish and the start of a career as Salimu, the older brother to Touwa did. Salimu commenced training to be a tailor. The nervous ones were those who wanted to continue with schooling. They worried over the many hurdles they had to overcome. The major hurdle was to pass the exam, coupled with the selection to get the few places available in upper primary schools. The ability of the parent to pay the school fees and the fear that after spending that much of the family's money on education, whether one would get a good job to help the family out of poverty. There were few opportunities for further progress on leaving school at standard four, while there were numerous training opportunities like teacher training, or a number of technical schools where various skills could be learned, after the upper primary school completion. All those chances depended on passing the year end exams and the rest was based on luck, which were the selection and the ability to pay school fees. Auntie Atanasia played a huge role in alleviating the many worries that Touwa had by her reassurance and financial support.

The constant studying, the frequent practice on past exam papers and the near a hundred percent attendance in school made the year appear very short and the exam days were fast approaching. Obviously there were high levels of nervousness that was made worse by the exam day factors. First, the pupils had to leave their familiar class surroundings to a new class in the nearby Nanjara Upper primary school. That school had a large one storey building that appeared huge to the pupils. The pupils had not been or seen at close-up a first floor of a building and to climb the stirs to the first floor, then enter a new class for examinations was exhausting. The teachers were also nervous because if a whole school failed it was a reflection of poor teaching while a higher pass was credit to the teaching staff.

The Head teacher asked each pupil to eat a light but very good meal on the morning of the examination. Touwa's sister and grandmother interpreted the good food as corn porridge with milk and sugar, a roast banana and a glass of fermented milk. With that food as breakfast, Touwa went to school to sit for his examination. At school the teachers were already distributing the new writing and geometry sets for the exam before the short walk to go to the exam venue at the Nanjara Upper primary school building. There was a deafening silence as the pupils walked a short distance to the exam room. The pupils stood in two lines facing the room for exams as the door was shut allowing examiners to do the room set up. At exactly 8.30 the door opened and the head teacher facing the pupils put their minds at peace by saying that there was nothing to worry about, as it was exactly as they had practiced. The pupils started going into the classroom. Just in front of Touwa a boy called Kalembo, made the first step and saw the desks. He dropped his pen; on picking it up, he again dropped his ruler. The nervousness was so high that he dropped the geometry set as he picked the ruler. To speed up getting into the class Touwa helped in picking up the many items of the geometry set and with the help of the teacher the pupil was helped to his assigned desk. He was given a new pen as the nib was broken.

At 09.00 hours, the order to start was given and the one hour of the examination became *'the moment.'* That was the moment when ones life path was set. It was therefore a moment of significance and importance that would shape the lives of many. In the evening after three sets of exam papers, the pupils went home in complete silence, avoiding the usual evening games of wrestling, football kicking, friendly *'ndulele'* fights, and the usual test of agility by running and jumping on the river stones and the show of strength when boys carry one another on their backs. There was no return to school after that day, as the teachers were busy with the lower classes that were also doing tests to move to higher classes; after which it was the start of the Christmas holidays.

Waiting for examination results was a distressing period as all plans were subject to the type of results obtained. On the results day almost all the pupils went to school to hear the results as read loudly by the Head teacher who only read the names of the selected pupils. He read the fifteen names very fast as there was a cry of elation by those who heard their names. When the names of Touwa and his friend Shirima were called the two friends hugged each other and found no word to express their happiness. Those who passed turned their attention to consoling those who failed and so that was the end of lower primary school education for Touwa. The next school was Kirongo Upper primary which was to start in the next two months in January. Salema's hope and wish was that Touwa passed and go to the upper primary school. Since that wish was granted, he started preparing in order to pay for the expensive needs that were to follow. He also realised that his son could read the books, improve his life and that of the whole family. That good feeling was slowly replacing the grief he endured at the beginning of the year. The rekindled friendship between Salema and his father Shenji also helped Salema to overcome his grief. Last but not least of the healing factors was Touwa's pass and selection Kirongo Upper Primary school. That was a boarding school, where there was better food, electricity, clean water and above all good learning atmosphere devoid of all the village problems. The cost was high, but Salema was delighted and determined to ensure his son, the first to attain that level of education should not be let down, a mutual feeling of father and son. The shoes, the uniform, the new towels, socks, articles the young boy had never possessed till then, were now essentials. Smiling with happiness Touwa was eager that the school term started sooner, in order for him to start using his new possessions.

That new school, Kirongo Upper Primary, was nine kilometres from home through a winding dusty road passable with difficulty during rainy season and very dusty during the dry season. That was the road Touwa travelled to and from his new school Kirongo Upper Primary School for the four years that followed.

CHAPTER 2

Stepping out from the village

Good-bye Nanjara school:

During that Christmas holiday, Touwa and his friend Shirima appeared visibly happy due to the thoughts of going away in January, not only stepping out of the village but actually leaving and staying away for a while. That was a period of the term time, which was six months without seeing their village mates or relatives. For Touwa he would not see his father, grandmother, grandad, brothers and his sister until the holiday break in June. The thoughts of getting new and better shoes uniforms, socks, clean bedding material, towels, and even a suitcase eclipsed all issues of loneliness that could be a result of being away from the family or homesickness which was then unknown. In his wisdom Touwa was probably right in thinking that he was going to better things than he was leaving behind as his grandad had told him. He was leaving behind the village chores that involved daily fetching of forage such as grass cutting, bundling and carrying home for the in house kept animals. Early morning herding the cattle to '*aulo*', the central meeting area where some village disputes were debated and solved. It was also where all the cattle were collected in the morning, to be moved to the forest to feed and the place where each cattle owner would collect their herd to take home in the evenings. Farm work, harvesting, wood fetching and chopping were just some of the many chores Touwa would then be exempt from carrying out. Touwa and Shirima regularly went to the river to scrub their hard skinned feet in anticipation of wearing shoes with socks. When they went to church on Sunday they saw the smart dressed boys and girls that attended Upper primary schools but they were too timid to ask them anything about their anticipated attendance to Upper primary school. While the two friends were wishing for January to come, their parents were frantic raising the money for school fees. Salema had to find the relatively large sums of money payable in advance for school fees. It was then he realised that he was not as rich as he thought. There were additions like pocket money, uniforms and travelling costs. Some friends were willing to lend Salema but some of the village folk thought that school fees was a waste of good earned cash and that school was unimportant since they were able to be rich without education. That attitude held by some of the village folk forced Salema to reduce the number of friends, choosing quality to quantity. He became a man with few friends because many were avoiding him, afraid he would borrow to educate his child and failing to repay. When Salema realised that people were keeping away from him lest he asked for some cash, he had to think big. The one big idea was to lease some land, part of his large farm to be paid in produce that he sold made cash and paid his debts. He also expanded the cultivated area of his farm using machinery like tractors and in so doing his cash flow was good and he met all his obligations. The school opening day was fast approaching. The fees were ready; the new shoes were polished, the uniforms were made and tried on by Touwa, ironed and placed in the wooden type box used as a suitcase ready for the journey.

The Kirongo upper Primary school:

It was very early on a Sunday morning when Touwa was to board a bus at Tarakea market to go to Kirongo Upper Primary School. It was the first time Touwa alone had to board a bus. His father Salema sensing his fear accompanied him in the bus to Usseri market place, from where Touwa would walk with his friends to the school a kilometre away. The bus was full, so full that it was even difficult to stand in the bus without being squeezed. The bus moved; it was slow at first, then it gathered speed leaving a wake of a dusty cloud behind. When Touwa looked through the window, he saw the trees moving very fast, but the amazing events did not end there as he saw two buses passing each other fast without one of them stopping as it was done in the village paths. To add to his fear he noted that the passing vehicles hurled dust to all the passengers making it almost impossible to see but the odd thing was that neither driver reduced their speeds nor showed concern despite a moment of no visibility. He was terrified at first but as his father was calm he knew it was safe. It was through that rugged dusty road that Touwa accompanied by his father travelled from the village of Nanjara to Usseri market place and eventually to Kirongo Upper primary school. At Usseri market place, Salema checked that his son had all that was demanded by the school namely clean pair of school uniform and other essentials like vests, pants, towels, soap, tooth brush and a jumper for the cold evenings as there were no log fires to provide warmth. Some pocket money to buy little luxuries like sweets was provided. Salema ensured the money for school fees was safe by putting it in Touwa's pocket, then pinned the pocket and gave the strictest instructions that he was to give that money to the headmaster and ensure a receipt was issued. That receipt was to be kept for six month when Touwa would return home during the half year break. When he was satisfied that all was well Salema shook his son's hand and asked him to join his friends to proceed to school. The group of boys from Nanjara and Tarakea looked elegant with their shoes, socks, khaki short trousers and white shirts. It was the first time they wore shoes, that was why they walked rather funny with their suitcases either on their heads or their shoulder. They passed a small area with tall trees where the forestry department conducted some experiments. Past the tall trees was a clear view of Kirongo Upper Primary school, which was built on the top of a steep hill. To reach the school however the pupils had to negotiate a steep gorge that was the remains of a long dried up ancient mighty river. At the bottom of the gorge was a small stream of flowing water. They had to cross by stepping on stones that were above the water level. That was a hurdle those boys had never encountered. The idea of jumping over the stones with shoes had never been attempted. Touwa and Shirima were experts in jumping over stones in crossing a river even much more rapid than that encountered at the Kirongo stream, but without shoes. The two boys knew they could cross the stream without shoes. With shoes and socks removed, the problem was solved and all crossed the stream without getting wet. A good artistic drawing showing a hand pointing the route to follow to Kirongo upper primary school was a sign post that was seen next after climbing up the steep gorge. After completing the climb, the hill top was flat with many school buildings. The senior pupils showed the new pupils where the dormitories, the classrooms including where all other school facilities were located. The dormitory was an old church which was partitioned into open plan rooms with beds for the pupils. There were shower room s and tap water although the toilets were the pit types but with water facilities to wash hands. After that tour, the allocation of beds was done; a bell rang, calling to assemble for dinner. It was the most mouth-watering dinner of rice and meat with a desert that was milk. That kind of good food had not been consumed at home in the village. After washing their utensils in the scullery, the friends went for a stroll to shake the full bellies to get some comfort. It was now dusk, the generators were started and there was light all around the school. It was so amazing seeing a little bulb that produced light more powerful than the kerosene lamps of home. At bedtime Touwa reflected on the day's events and remembered his grandad's words to always aspire for better things, and then he drifted to a sound sleep.

The bell rang; it was Monday morning, a signal to wake up, wash and get ready for breakfast. Tea, bread with butter and jam, that was almost heaven, as the two friends Touwa and Shirima commented. The bell rang; it was for assembly and inspection before entry to the classrooms. Like in the lower primary school, assembly involved the hygiene inspection, which was a check for combed hair, wash face and behind the ears, brush teeth, cut and washed nails. The uniform had to be clean and well pressed. That was not a problem for standard five classes, as all their clothes were new. The pupils entered into their new classroom and chose where to sit. All stood up at once with a loud greeting: *'Good morning sir'* as the teacher entered the class. That was the start of standard five classes in the Upper primary school at Kirongo.

The lessons were conducted in one hour intervals after which a bell signalling a lesson change was sounded, and then another teacher would enter the class for a different lesson as per timetable unlike the lower primary school. It was at the end of the day when the pupils realised the big difference in the learning in upper primary school. There were more lessons, each lesson had a different teacher, and the pupils could not imagine there were so much more to learn including new subjects they had not heard before. There were also more activities like football that was played in a bigger, better and smoother field, sports like running, high jump and long jump. Hobbies were introduced like gardening, and fish keeping and a chance to join the scout club, for girls it was 'girl guides'. The many activities made the school a good community especially for those who lived within the school as boarders. Those activities also were a setting for a great chance to acquire new friends. To alleviate home sickness the boarders were allowed to go home at some weekends or parents would visit to give some more pocket money or brothers or sisters would visit just to see the school. All those activities made the first six months at Kirongo Upper primary school pass without incidents of worry or home sickness. At the end of the term there were examinations and grading that showed the level each pupil was ranked in the classroom. The first three always got a reward, a pen, pencil, book or any academic enhancing article. That was the main topic when a pupil went home, the parents would ask of ones position out of the forty pupils of a class. Shirima was always ranked from first to fifth but Touwa was a bit lower from fifth to tenth. No one wanted to be number forty, as that meant that one's average in the lessons was the lowest. In some cases all the pupils could have passes but the ranking was to encourage competition, which stimulated hard working and raised the aspiration to pass to an excellent level and not to be satisfied with just a pass. The last bell on that Friday after the exam results signified the start of holiday time when Touwa and Shirima packed and left on that Friday evening. It was a rainy Friday evening, and the two boys started walking to the Usseri market place where they could catch a bus or a lorry to take them home.

A holiday meant going home:

It was a rainy Friday evening; all vehicles that left Moshi town were late as travelling through the slippery roads was slower than on the dry roads. It was luck that an uncle of Touwa, named Katarimo, who had a passenger vehicle was driving a full bus. He was a clever traveller who used chains on the tyres and could travel on muddy roads. When he saw Touwa he told him to jump into the bus including Shirima as Touwa could not leave his friend behind. The bus started to move. It was a small bus for twenty eight passengers but on a guess there could be fifty passengers that squeezed against each other sitting and standing. The journey gradually became more comfortable as some passengers alighted giving a little space to breathe. On the last kilometre or two from Tarakea, the rains were heavier the road more slippery, and even with the chains on the tyres the bus stuck in the mud. The conductor asked all to get out and help to push. Touwa and Shirima who had a free ride in the uncle's bus had to volunteer to push. The shoes that were highly polished, the brilliant white shirts and the immaculately ironed shorts experienced mud spatter and great amount of dirt for the first time in six months. As they helped to push the bus the tyres sprayed mud to the cleanest boys from head to toe. They knew they were back at home as the dirt was a memory of the past days in the village. They could not be seen like that by anyone. They were upper primary school boys; they had to shine to their best. As soon as they reached their drop zone they got out passed by river Tarakea, washed in the cold evening stream water, changed their attire and proceeded home to meet their family. It became a proper home coming with clean clothes showing a better example to their younger siblings and a good impression to their parents.

On his way home Touwa passed by his grandfather who became very excited to see him. On arriving home his grandmother and his sister Mkaleso were also very excited and happy while elder brother Salimu just casually commented: *'so you are back to help with work here'*, as he introduced his wife Mamasawe to his younger brother. Touwa did not understand the attitude of his older brother. According to a

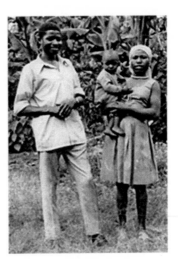

Salimu and wife mamasawe

brief by Ndesumbuka, there was no longer a happy family after the untimely death of Mkasu; after that time Salema kept away from the Nanjara farm and spent more time in the boundary farm. Salimu became arrogant as no one could tell him what to do, using his new freedom to oppress the younger siblings, doing very little work, with excessive socializing and drinking of *'mbege'*. The work was left to his sister Mkaleso and grandmother Yohana including his younger bothers Melikoi and Tabu. Mamasawe and Salimu were the bosses who worked very little pushed the little ones Melikoi and Tabu to work so hard that Mkaleso could no longer tolerate their misuse of power. Mkaleso left home to live with her boyfriend Kiberenge, after a serious quarrel with Salimu. Yohana was strong enough to look after Tabuni, the youngest sibling but could not also care for the animals and the *'shamba'*. *(Shamba means the small plot where food crops are grown).* There was evidence of neglect, as weeds grew everywhere, bananas were not spaced or shaved clean, coffee was not pruned and the compound looked unclean. Shenji and Yohana did not like the deterioration of the premises. In order to correct and reverse the trend of decay they called a meeting of all the elders. Shenji the grandpa informed Salema, Makinafu Makimaina, Kimosoyo, Anyika, Sirikwa and other elders of the village, who settled the matter by giving Salimu a fine, which was a goat to slaughter and two barrels of *'mbege'*. Salema was furious as he heard the catalogue of abuse; he took Melikoi and Tabu to the boundary farm.

Early in the morning Shenji came roaring as usual to wake up his grandson Touwa. He announced with pride that later on there was a goat to be slaughtered to celebrate his grandson's home coming. Salema was called to enjoy with his sons. The short family feast was enjoyed by all. All the younger brothers were happy to see Touwa who had grown a lot as he had eaten better food in the boarding school. All the elders, that is, grandfather and grandma including Salema were very excited at Touwa's home coming. Touwa liked to keep the areas around the huts clean by sweeping and removing any growth along the pathways as he had learned in school. Grandfather was so excited that he gave an order that elder brother should not force Touwa to do the grass cutting or foraging for animal feeds. Touwa however was willing and helped with the home chores as he was not a lazy boy despite protection from grandad. During the holiday period Touwa spent lots of days with his father at the boundary farm. Touwa noticed that his father was not as happy as before he first left for school but he was too young to ask. The events that were happening at home were related to Touwa by his younger brother Ndesumbuka who told him of their father's unhappiness that was due to Salimu's behaviour and the loss of Mkasu. That information was supported with the fact that Salema never visited the Nanjara home except when called by his father. He called the Nanjara home 'manyumbu'. According to Salema 'nyumbu' was one of the most stupid animals in the wilderness; it hardly defended or protected one another against being eaten by lions. Despite being a cheap source of meat, lions were selective as they ate 'nyumbu' only when food was very scarce as their meat was not

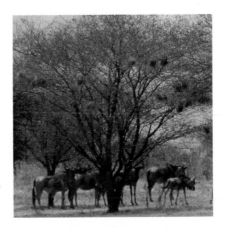

Wilderbist (Nyumbu)

palatable. *'Manyumbu'* therefore meant *'fools'* a *term* directed to Salimu and all his friends. Salema was angry with Salimu, his first son, because he had left the proceeds of the estate to Salimu to help with the upkeep of the younger children but Salimu used all the money from the sale of coffee and other farm produce for his own socializing and drinking. The continuation of this discord led to the deterioration of the education of many of his younger brothers especially Ndesumbuka who was then close to completing his lower primary education. The arrival of Touwa, his smartness, his growth and his continuous politeness help to make Salema happy. The celebration that followed was an enjoyable moment for Salema and his children; Salimu, Mkaleso, Touwa, Ndesumbuka, Melikoi, Tabu and Tabuni. It was harvesting period; very busy time for everyone, that made the holiday appear short. As the holiday was coming to an end, Salema was working at a fast pace to find and assemble the required fees and expenditure money.

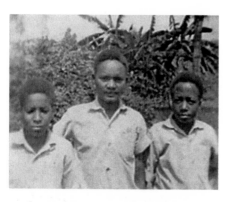

Mkwe and friends at Kirongo

On the leaving day Touwa was happy to receive the money for school fees that he pinned in the pocket as before and was glad to leave the then sad home, and the hope that the brothers would soon leave and follow him. The five months that followed, the routine and life at Kirongo

Upper Primary School was the same, comfortable and conducive to learning. New friends like Tairo and Ludo made life at school for Touwa a happy moment. It was only when Touwa remembered his younger brothers at home that he became sad knowing the cause of their unhappiness was the passing on of their beloved mother who was the rock of the family compounded by the rude attitude of the elder brother towards their father. Touwa hoped that on his return in November, at the end of the term, life at home would have changed to a happier one. Touwa was returning home with good news that he had passed to go to standard six. It was a rainy afternoon that the boarding pupils were free to go home. With their belongings in a small suitcase Touwa and his friend Shirima set out to go home. All transport was paralysed as the roads were too slippery even for vehicles with chained wheels. The two boys longed to reach home so they kept the suitcases at a friend close to the school and started walking the nine kilometres to their homes. That tough journey was to prove that the two friends Shirima and Touwa had a strong bond as they helped each other to cross swollen streams due to excessive rains. Touwa arrived home, first to greet grandad who expressed warmth and love then to his brother's hut to find a muted welcome even on revealing he had passed to go to standard six. Yohana, the grandma, Tabuni, the little boy, Salimu and his wife

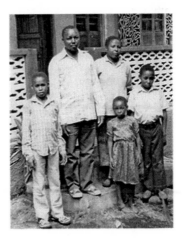

Mkaleso and family

Mamasawe were the only residents in the Nanjara home. Mkaleso (pictured with her family)had moved and was establishing her family with Tarimo her husband. She appeared happy and contented but unhappy with the changes that had occurred in the home she left. Ndesumbuka, Melikoi and Tabu were all in the boundary farm with Salema, their father. The home coming of Touwa was a reason to celebrate according to Shenji. The next day after making the compound tidy, Touwa left to see his father at the boundary farm, eager to meet with his brothers. Ndesumbuka was old enough to know a bit of the village gossip, the talk that helped Touwa to know what went on in the village. The boundary farm was no longer a bush but had developed to a good village, Salema had neighbours like Lenkoya, Ole Kilusu, Ole Parpaai, Mseseve Mangoroho, Karioki and Doiki used to meet to enjoy drinks like *'mbege'* or *'kangara'* an alcoholic drink made with honey, that Salema had learned to make from his new friends. Life was near normal, as there was the usual socializing, children playing, making toys, going and coming from schools.

Salema hated the deterioration of his Nanjara home that he called *'Manyumbu'*. He did not even go to visit wife Alina but he was working hard as he was then a single parent taking care of the late Mkasu's boys. There was a lot of work in the farms that included weeding the young crop plants to take hold and grow healthily. Touwa worked hard in the fields to impress his father and to earn his school fees. The holiday passed without any family crisis, and that was good, as Touwa left for school that January morning.

On arrival at Kirongo Upper primary school Touwa felt proud to have the chance of showing new pupils the facilities of the school, as he was shown the previous year, noticing how nervous they were. In standard six there was no significant change of lessons, the only new activity was the eligibility to join the scouts. Touwa became a scout. The camp fires and singing were the best things Touwa experienced and loved. The excitement that the scout movement provided, school became a happy place to be and the years passed quickly.

As the years passed at Kirongo:

Many changes were expected as the country became independent. All school children received a plastic cup, to celebrate the country's Independence Day or *'uhuru'* day. With independence came many changes. There were country wide and family changes that Touwa had to get abreast with. Ndesumbuka would write to Touwa to tell of the changes happening in the family. In one of the letters, Salimu the older brother had a daughter and it did not take long before news that the Salema acquired a wife and that a sister or brother would add to their count. It was not long as another letter announced the birth of a child, a girl, who was named Mamnana. Soon there were so many births that Touwa lost count as he was aspiring to pass his standard eight exams to get selection to secondary school.

Touwa was worried of failure as shared by his friends pictured above that was Ludo (centre)and Tairo, left side of Ludo. Personally Touwa had added problems. The home to go to was not a happy place, and if he passed the school fees were so high that his father could not afford and if he tried to pay it would be at the expense of his younger brothers who would hot have the chance of ever getting an upper primary school education. In his wisdom Touwa decided to apply to a seminary where he would get a secondary education free, and possibly be a priest. His father's reaction to his son's aspiration to be priest was a definite 'no'. Touwa's application to a seminary was accepted but he was afraid to go against his father's wishes. There was a change announced by the government that made Touwa's dilemma less important. The new government announced some education changes. To the ears of all parents in the land, came the news that brought happiness: *'School fees were abolished; no fees were needed for education in primary or secondary schools'.* Touwa like all other pupils aspired to pass as the fees issue was solved.

From each Upper primary school, only a small number were selected to go to secondary school. That government announcement, made clear the opportunities ahead, as the stumbling block, the school fees was removed. All pupils were very nervous days before and after exams. After the last paper, the Headmaster gave permission for all to go home. It was the last day in that school. The pupils were told to check for results after three weeks. Touwa and his friend Shirima packed all their belongings in their small wooden suitcases and left for home. On meeting his grandad, Touwa was almost tearful with the worry of failure, but grandad as usual cheered him up by giving him a sweet calabash of 'mbege' and said, *'you can read, write and speak a new language, you are educated and to me you can do anything you like so stop crying.'* Touwa felt comforted by those words and with the additional effect of *'mbege'* he relaxed. Everyone he visited asked how he felt after finishing school, as many village folk did not know that there was more education after upper primary school.

Early in the morning Shenji came to wake up Touwa and to check whether he was happier. Shenji liked to make his grandchildren happy by then giving something nice to eat. That time it was a chicken boiled in flavours with onions and tomatoes in thick gravy, eaten with roast and boiled bananas. The youngest brother Tabuni was then aged five would associate such good welcome home treats with going to school. Touwa and Shirima spent their time by talking, visiting families and waiting for the three tense weeks to get results. The day for the results was announced in church. Touwa and Shirima travelled the nine kilometres to hear the results at Kirongo, but there was no one in the school. The two boys like many others returned home still worried. There was a determination to travel every day to hear the results. It was a Thursday afternoon when the boys arrived at Kirongo Upper primary school to find the results announced. Some were happy but those who did not see their names slowly walked and went home. The happy ones were in groups chatting happily. Touwa was so scared to go to the notice board but when Shirima came towards Touwa from the notice boards he looked sad and Touwa's heart sunk. Shirima said to Touwa, *'you have passed and I failed'* Shirima's name was not on the board but Touwa passed and he was going to Umbwe Secondary school, a place to spend the 9th to the 12th year of school that was termed forms one to four. Rather than joining the pass group Touwa followed his friend who was crying to comfort him and together they went home. As soon as they parted Touwa went straight to tell his grandad, and then speeded to the boundary farm to tell his dad of the news. Salema was happy as he knew the burden of school fees was lifted. Brothers Ndesumbuka, Melikoi and Tabu expressed their happiness. Salema's new wife Mamoroi was worried that Salema's money would be spent on Touwa and his younger brothers for their education. Salema ordered a sheep to be slaughtered to prove that he was very happy and that he was prepared to support Touwa to continue with his education. Touwa's Christmas holiday in 1964 appeared short as he was very busy. The school uniform was black long trousers, white shirt, black leather shoes. Other items of clothing included warm jumper and a pair of white sheets. The school provided blankets. Salema and Touwa travelled to Moshi town. It was all an excitement to Touwa who had never ventured so far from home. The road was still rugged as he travelled towards Moshi. He saw large bridges, deeper river gorges, and bigger rivers than Tarakea. Closer to Moshi town, the road became very smooth with no bumps with the numerous vehicles large and small travelling at speeds Touwa had never imagined. The road was wider and smoother as the bus approached to

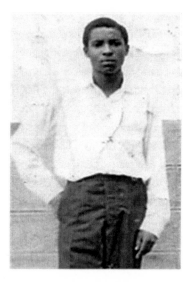

Touwa at 15 at Umbwe

Moshi town that had so many cars forcing the bus driver to reduce speed. According to Touwa, Moshi town was huge with buildings that were taller than his father's cypress trees. Touwa imagined telling his younger brothers about his travels. There were more trips to Moshi town, sixty kilometres away, to buy the essentials to enable Touwa to travel and study at Umbwe Secondary school.

CHAPTER 3

Farther away from home

Umbwe Secondary school was eighty kilometres from Nanjara, on the western side of the slopes of Mount Kilimanjaro. Touwa had neither heard of it nor had the least idea of where it was. It was a letter from the Headmaster of Umbwe Secondary school that revealed the detail route on how to reach there from Moshi town. Salema was proud, he bought all that the new school required and even more. Touwa was ecstatic but the thought of leaving his best friend Shirima behind was a subject of concern. He was driven to know that he was going for better things as his granddad had said.

New school with great expectations:

On one cool January morning, the fifteen year old boy, Touwa set to travel eighty kilometres to his new school accompanied by his father to Moshi town. At the busy, noisy, dusty and congested Moshi town bus stop, Touwa met other new students on their way to Umbwe. Salema was satisfied that Touwa had friends and together they could take another bus to Umbwe. The mini bus to Umbwe was full or rather closely packed, but the aspiration to see Umbwe Secondary school was so great that not even one of the passengers uttered a word of complaint. The bus stop was about half a kilometre from the school gates, so all students had to alight, and carrying their suitcases walked to see the majestic buildings of Umbwe Secondary school. The school consisted of classrooms, the laboratories, the staff offices that appeared to enclose the dormitories where all the students would sleep. From building to building there was a well defined walking path levelled and cemented with a roof that would protect students and teachers from rain as they walk from one classroom to another. The rest of the school compound was covered with well maintained lawn. There were flower beds that gave the school an air of sophistication and beauty. There was a Church, football, badminton, basketball and volleyball fields. A well built professional lawn tennis court was the pride of the school. The toilets unlike those at Kirongo were not pit ones but water cleaned systems that all first year (form-one) students had to be shown their proper usage. Like in upper primary school there was a bell sound to call one, to do or to go elsewhere. That bell at 5pm was calling for dinner. The dinner, rice and meat with fruits afterwards that was scrumptious. At 7 pm the bell was for assembly to be given information about the school by the duty master, who explained the available facilities and how to get access to many of the school activities with the emphasis on the rules on what could or could not be done while one was a student at Umbwe. That was a Sunday evening, and at ten all the students had to be in their dormitories as the generator that produced electricity was switched off. In his bed, Touwa reflected on the extra ordinary day that started in his village of Nanjara, the travelling, the new friends, new school and the prospect of starting form one class in the morning. As he remembered his granddad's words that he was going to better things, he drifted quietly to sleep.

The bell rang again, that was six am, time to wash, dress, and go for breakfast then inspection at 7 am. At inspection the class master would check cleanliness, dress code and attendance check. Lessons would begin at 7.30am prompt and timetables were adhered to strictly. The class of thirty five form-one students with their brilliant white shirts, well ironed black trousers entered the classroom to start the four years of schooling, to get a GCSE (General Certificate of School Education)also known as O-level Certificate of Education. It was a January morning in 1965 when Touwa entered a class of thirty five students that was termed form-one. The teachers were from different nations and races, black and white Americans, Irish, British, Tanzanians and Kenyans. It was the first time Touwa made a close contact with a person whose skin was not as dark as his. It was an experience that he saved for six months to tell his family. All lessons were conducted in English. Many of the teachers could not speak Swahili the lingua franca for all the people of Tanzania that was adopted as a National language soon after independence. The changes that the new independent government brought were streaming out fast.

After the school fees removal policy, came the self help policy, the integration policy and the universal primary education for all.

The universal primary education meant that pupils would study up to standard seven, and then do examinations for secondary education entrance, instead of the previous standard four. That meant primary education as it was then referred to, would not take eight years but only seven, after which it would become a secondary education.

The integration policy meant that students going to secondary schools would be a mix from many regions, many religions and many ethnic groups and would be eligible to go to any school they chose whether government school or faith schools. Umbwe was a faith school of the Catholic faith but it was taking students with a variety of faith backgrounds. The form-one class consisted of students from a variety of faiths and ethnic affiliations but all looked similar with their uniforms. As the days passed, the students started to know one another and friendships were formed that submerged all ethnic and religious apparent differences.

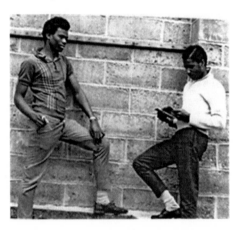

Touwa at Umbwe with Mboro

The self help policy meant that students in all schools should take part in cost reduction by doing manual work that would eliminate employing cleaners, gardeners and technicians for minor repairs. That was translated by schools that students kept all the school clean from classrooms to toilets, tidiness from lawn upkeep to flowers tendering and janitor duties.

Lessons were basically as those in primary school but more in detail and sophistication with added new subjects like the branches of science, namely Biology, Chemistry and Physics with the various branches of Mathematics like Geometry, Statistics and Calculus. There were laboratories where science principles were demonstrated and where students were shown how to do some experiments to prove scientific facts. After the lessons in the classrooms there were extra curriculum activities that included sports, games, self help assignments, and competitions that earned points for each dormitory with a good prize for the winners. In the evening after dinner there was a two hour mandatory study time after which the generator was off and it was obviously bed time as the whole place was as dark as the village of Nanjara. The many activities of

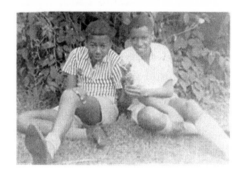

Touwa at Umbwe with Linus

the school occupied Touwa's time, as he enjoyed playing lawn tennis and football. It was only in bed when he had time for his usual reflections. It was then that he would remember home, his father, brothers, sister and grandma. Above all, he would speculate on the things his grandpa would do or say the next time he went home. That was the way school life was followed throughout the four years at Umbwe with minor adjustments on the third and fourth years.

Going home was a holiday:

The six months of the first term at Umbwe were hectic; at the end of that term Touwa was on the way home to visit his relatives. He was taller, healthier and looked very smart. His father was proud to see him and granddad planned the usual welcome when all the family met to talk to Touwa. Due to the death of Mkasu, Touwa's mother, and the uncaring attitude of Salimu, the progress in education of the younger brothers to Touwa especially Ndesumbuka was hampered, as Ndesumbuka was still in lower primary school. He had flour more years to complete basic primary education, which was standard seven, in accordance to the new education changes. Melikoi, spent most of his time with a teacher called Ngaile whose residence had rooms to spare for use by those in need. That enabled Melikoi to be in a better learning environment and escape the turmoil of the family. Touwa started to get to know his step mother number two or the third wife of Salema. There was a mutual respect but not love between the wife, Mamoroi, and Touwa. Touwa remembered his mother's request to Yohana and wondered whether that new woman would treat or care for his brothers well. Salema appeared happy as his family or rather his new family was getting on well. He had some money then as he did not have to pay any school fees. Touwa divided his holiday, spending time with grandma and grandpa and improving Salema's first house to use as his residence during holidays. Kimwai who was as old as Salimu was Touwa's uncle who helped and advised Touwa to improve the residence to make it as good as the school dormitory. Kimwai became the best friend to Touwa as they could talk about everything especially the changes Touwa observed as his was becoming a teenager. It was Kimwai who reunited Touwa

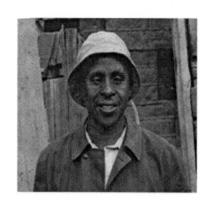

Uncle Kimwai

and Shirima who at that time was repeating the standard seven in preparation for Secondary school entry examinations.

When the holiday period was coming to its final days, Touwa wished Shirima success and promised that their friendship was intact. Kimwai always trimmed Touwa's hair to ensure a smart look on return to school. Touwa was busy, he was going to many of the relatives, the notable one was the auntie Atanasia, his mother's younger sister, and who always gave some money, advice, heartfelt love and goodwill. The final journey was to see his father for some travelling money and other expenses. No one understood why Salema gave the money to his wife Mamoroi to give to Touwa but what followed was a clear signal the there was no love for Mkasu's children in that new family, as Mamoroi put the money on the floor instead of giving to Touwa. Salema was embarrassed, he picked up the money, and gave to his son, saying *you go to your school with no worries* as he realised the level of Mamoroi's feelings towards Mkasu's children. Touwa was old enough to understand that reaction of hostility, but remained composed and polite by saying thank you to Mamoroi for letting him have the money. Touwa said farewell to his father, brothers and with a smile to Mamoroi, left for his second term at Umbwe.

Touwa's beloved auntie—Atanasia:

Mkasu, Touwa's mother was from a polygamous family. She was a fourth child of a second wife. Mkasu's mother had six children, a boy, the first born was Melikoi, followed by all girls namely; Mamshimbi, Mamkwe, Mkasumaili (Mkasu), Candida and Atanasia. Atanasia was married to Masika, a well to do gentleman

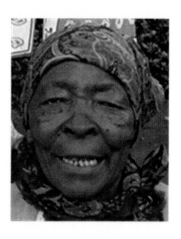

Atanasia the auntie to Touwa

who had a lorry, a sign of wealth. They lived close to the local dispensary which was also a route to and from school during the early period of Touwa's school days. The kindness of the auntie encouraged Touwa to pass there for something to eat when he was going or coming from school. Auntie Atanasia treated Touwa with love and was keen to ensure Touwa had eaten. That kindness of Atanasia continued during the periods of lower primary school to secondary education. That bond and kindness was in memory that was kept in Touwa's mind all the time. One memorable occasion was when Touwa was at Umbwe Secondary school when he went to see his auntie to tell her that he was going back to school. When the auntie checked her purse and found she had no money to give to Touwa, she apologised and asked if Touwa would do something for her. Touwa enthusiastically accepted. Touwa then followed his auntie to the grain store. Auntie Atanasia filled a large sack with grains and asked Towa to take it to the shop to sell. Touwa was glad to be able to do something for his auntie. He did not care whether his brilliant white shirt would get stained as he carried the sack on his shoulders and walked speedily to the shop. When he returned with a lot of money and the sack to auntie, she just said *'that is your pocket money to go to school'.* For a child who had no mother, that gesture made Touwa experience a kind of love as close as what a mother could give. It was those moments that made living in the green pastures of home memorable, relaxing, and happy and it was that gave the urge to return to those green pastures when Touwa was away.

The life while at Umbwe:

Like many of his fellow students Touwa took part in many extra curriculum activities like football and athletics. He was selected a team member for his house team that competed for prizes. Touwa learned the rules that enabled him to take part in playing the games of football, table tennis, lawn tennis, volleyball and badminton. It was in a two hundred metre sprint that Touwa excelled to a level to represent his school in some competitions. Those numerous activities at Umbwe, including taking swimming lessons, meant there were no times to complain of boredom.

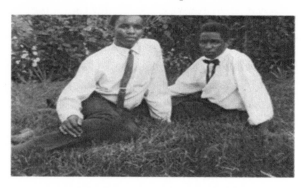

Touwa with Shirima at Secondary school

The holidays that followed became the most relaxing holidays because Touwa's best friend Shirima had passed and selected to go to Old Moshi secondary school. That meant the two friends would travel together most of the journeys to their schools which were both close to Moshi town. Life for Touwa during the holidays was the daily help in the family chores. Touwa was proud to chop wood for his grandmother, Yohana, cleaned and swept the compound around his house, an act that pleased Shenji, the granddad. Kimwai, who was working as a forest guard encouraged Touwa to go to see what he did. He was a mentor to Touwa as he taught him how to plant seedlings and saw seeds for germination. On Sundays, however, Touwa and Shirima would go to their friends where they would socialise by exchanging of stories from other secondary schools, drinking *'mbege'* and usually dancing. The friends that finished their school at standard four were now young men with only one ambition, to get married, unlike Touwa and Shirima, who had one ambition that was to see what that extra schooling would bring. With Shirima starting form one and Touwa entering form two; life was not so different for the two friends. During term time school work was paramount but during the holidays social events dominated the activities. That extra social life needed some cash.

Uncle Kimwai arranged for Touwa and Shirima to get a job at his forest nursery centre to water the germinating seeds. The extra cash helped Touwa to improve his father's house by laying a concrete floor. It was an improvement that was admired by all. New clothes made Touwa and Shirima stand out, they became a social attraction giving speeches and organising party events. That dancing and drinking caught Salema's attention as he thought that his son was getting to love the village life and ignore his school. He was furious. He refused to give pocket money and travel expenses money for use to go to school when asked. Touwa knew that his activities were not that good. He went to see granddad to tell how and why Salema was angry. Granddad called his son Salema to order him to issue the funds as he was sure Touwa would not go back to the village life. Although Salema was not happy with that order, he complied with it and Touwa showed respect by buying him a present the next time he was paid.

Ndesumbuka's plight:

The home problems fuelled partly by Salimu made Salema an unhappy man. His anger with Salimu, his first son was reflected in the treatment of the younger siblings. The pressure of having more children with the new wife was also a factor. The demands from wife number two who

99

was not promoted to number one after the death of Mkasu and the friction of the two wives may have eroded Salema's happiness. Ndesumbuka was finishing standard seven and Salema made no preparations for his progress. When Ndesumbuka completed primary education, he was not selected to go to a secondary school. Salema had assumed that the boy would just end his school days, but for the effort of Doiki a village councillor and a friend of Salema. Doiki's duties as a councillor were to check school progress, an opportunity that he got to know Ndesumbuka who was bright pupil and always passed well in the school tests. It took some convincing by Doiki and a teacher named Salekio that Salema accepted to support further schooling for Ndesumbuka. After the agreement that the boy needed more education, Salema with a letter from Salekio travelled with Ndesumbuka, through seven kilometres of bushy and hilly country to arrive at Illasit Full Primary school. That was in Kenya, it was difficult for Ndesumbuka but he was admitted into standard six for only two months where he proved himself by passing to go to standard seven the following year and eventually left with a pass and selection to Olkejuado Secondary School in Kenya which was a fee paying school. That was progress for his son that made Salema a happy man again at his boundary farm. Salema decided to find the school fees for his son to go to school in Kenya as he did not get the free education opportunity in Tanzania. The social circle for Salema increased but was different from that he left at *'Manyumbu'*. In this new social circle were Lenkoya, Mangoroho, Waha, Mseseve, Kariokii, Ole Parpaai, Ndeseya, and Ole Kilusu. The new group socialized by drinking *'kangara'* and *'mbege'*. Salema's happiness was almost complete as Ndesumbuka and Tabu were following the footsteps Touwa was taking. The fact that

Touwa was coming home reporting that he had passed and was going to other schools may have had negative effects as Touwa was still demanding help after eight years. Some school mates of Touwa were earning and supporting their families. Salema however still supported Touwa. Shenji, the granddad did not understand the education system but as he noted Touwa coming home smart and cleaner than any of the village folk he knew Touwa was out for better things and he gave a hundred percent support and encouragement, even when Salema was not too sure. During holidays Touwa earned some money and he was becoming financially independent of his father to a high extent in order to allow the possibility of education for the younger siblings.

Towards the GCSE exams:

On his last holiday before his O-level examinations, Touwa left home, said good—bye to his father, step mothers, brothers, his sister and the younger step brothers and sisters, without realizing that it was the last time he would spend more than two weeks in the village. It was also the last time Ndesumbuka, Melikoi and Tabu would be together with their father at the same time in the village. At Umbwe, studying for the O-level examinations was paramount. There was the compulsory two hours of mandatory study period. During that period the thirty five classmates studied seriously. After ten, all were supposed to be in bed to sleep, but some went to some small rooms and continued studying with candle light for an extended period until sleep overcomes. It was that level of hard work that dominated the last term at Umbwe Secondary school. That was 1968, when Touwa completed secondary education.

After the o-level examinations, it was a holiday, also the time to wait for results that were announced in the National newspaper. It was time to say good-bye to many friends like Linusi and Mboro.

A letter to cousin Mtele was rewarded with a reply that was also an invite to Mwadui Diamond mines where he worked. That journey was estimated to be 800 kilometres away from the village and it would take about 24 hours of travel through mostly rough, rugged and dusty roads. It was the first time Touwa was anticipating to venture so far away from his village and from Kilimanjaro Mountain and above all that, travelling on his own.

Chapter 4

Away from Kilimanjaro

An outward bound holiday:

The end of the term was also the end of four years of secondary school education that was concluded by the O-level examinations as they were popularly known. It was the start of a long wait for examination results. The results would determine a future that was better than that of primary education but there was the usual worry of the unknown. It was also the first time in all the eight years at boarding schools that Touwa was going on a holiday away from home instead of the homebound journey. The outward bound journey was away from home, Nanjara, away from the region, Kilimanjaro and onwards toward Mwadui Diamond mines. The journey to Mwadui Diamond mines was a planned visit to his cousin Mtele who was working as an engineer at the mines. That first travel undertaking for Touwa, outside Kilimanjaro was full of surprises. Touwa actually was physically in the towns that he had learned in Geography. He passed through Arusha, Manyara, Babati, Singida, and Nzega to Shinyanga. The mines were about fifty kilometres from

Shinyanga town. There were small villages and towns that were not even shown in Geography books. Touwa observed that unlike Kilimanjaro, the land was sparsely populated and that vegetation and the landscape were different from that of his home town and village. After travelling only a 100 kilometres from Moshi, his home town, he could not see the Kilimanjaro Mountain any more. There were a number of languages spoken from area to another but Kiswahili was always the dominant language. The huts were different; the crops for food were different, not the same as in Touwa's village. On arrival at Mwadui diamond mines, Mtele was there to welcome Touwa. The Mwadui diamond mine was an enclosed self sustaining village in the middle of a wilderness with water, electricity, housing, shops, and welfare systems that provide some commodities like milk, bread and meat at preferable discounted prices. The planned short visit was rewarded by Touwa securing a job at the lower security section of the mines, at a water purification plant working as a water quality tester. The work involved regular check of levels of chlorine and water clarity, recording and reporting as necessary. Mtele was very happy with Touwa for doing a job well and receiving good commendations on completion.

Time passed quick as Touwa was happy while working at the purification plant, giving little thought to the exam results until the newspapers and radios announced the results From the paper Touwa read that he had passed well and was selected to go to a high school, Usagara Secondary and High school in Tanga, a sea side municipality by the Indian Ocean. Touwa had two weeks to report to the new school. The first step was a prompt preparation to leave Mwadui for Nanjara to give the good news to his family.

The high school:

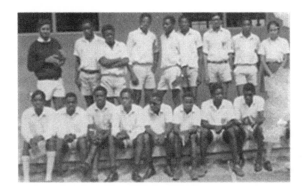

At High school

The journey back to Nanjara from Mwadui, was a happy
one for two reasons that Touwa had passed and was going
away again and he was financially secure as he bought all
he needed to go to his new school. He proved to his father
that he was independent by buying Salema a pair of shoes
by guessing his foot size. Salema was so proud when he put
on the shoes that fitted well. It was the first signs of rewards
for investing in his child's education that Salema noted.
It was probably those first signs that motivated Salema to
try educating all his children without exception. He took
a grim view of those who refused to pursue education in
their life's progress. As Touwa left for Usagara High School
after a week's visit to his family, Ndesumbuka and Tabu
were studying well and aspiring to go to secondary school
in the next one and three years respectively. The short visits
to his family, during holidays were not enough for Touwa
to know much of what was happening in the village like
the birth of new siblings, marriages of close relatives or
the intense friendship that had developed between Shenji

whose age was then 101 and his son Salema who was then 48 years old.

The travelling to Usagara School was by a steam train with speeds that never exceeded 30 kilometres per hour and that stopped in at every major and minor station. The journey of 300 kilometres took 24 hours but it was far from being boring but full of excitement, as each stop was a new town seen for the first time. The journey revealed different landscapes, the new mountains new variety of plants, new people and a marked temperature change. The temperatures were higher than those at Touwa's village. There was less need for blankets or pullovers but the need for mosquito nets. At Tanga railway station, the passengers mostly students got out as it was the end of the line. The residential accommodation and the school were walking distances from the station. At the residence the new fifth form met, introductions were made and new friendships formed. Usagara School was a day school not a boarding school like Umbwe, and it was for girls and boys. The only boarding students were the high school classes who were from outside Tanga town. The fifth and sixth form students were 70 in total and only 50 were boarders. The high school specialised in teaching Maths, Physics and Chemistry. The Headmaster Mr Marijani was a fast speaking, fast walking gentleman who was kind and gentle but portrayed a fierce and strict nature, a good quality that suited him as a Headmaster. The first term at Usagara School was spent by understanding the detailed level of study needed, getting used to studying with girls, getting to know the municipality of Tanga and the meeting different students and formation of friendships. During the June break, Touwa was lucky to get a job at a sisal processing and export company in Tanga, working in the records office. With the holiday spent working, Touwa had only a week to visit his relatives at Nanjara. It was in one of the visits to Nanjara through Moshi town that Touwa met a young man by the name of Lazaro who became a very close friend. It was later revealed by Salema that Lazaro and Touwa were first cousins and not only friends. The two friend's mothers had the same father but different mothers, that is, they were step sisters. Lazaro worked in a factory in Moshi town making it possible for the friends to meet during Touwa's travels.

News of the United States aspiring to send a man to the moon was constantly heard in the local radio. On his way to Tanga, returning to school after the holiday, in a slow steam train on the 21 July 1969, news of moon landing, and the voice of Neil Armstrong was broadcasted and was received by all passengers with jubilation through small hand held battery radios.

The two years at Usagara secondary and high school passed very quickly as the work load was a lot, such that there was little time devoted to extra curriculum activities, except for rare occasions of a football or a cricket match just before evening meals. As a high school student, Touwa took part in giving home tutorials to O-level certificate aspirants and evening classes for adults, in order to earn some pocket money. During holidays he worked in the Sisal Exporting Board in the records office with a good record that earned him repeat job acceptances. The last term at sixth form, there were lots of activities that signified the end of school and start of a profession.

Guidance was given to students on the merits of going to University, technical colleges or directly into paid jobs. Mr Marijani, the headmaster, was the mentor on how to make the appropriate applications. He gave advice based on the ability of the applicant. He knew the academic strength of each student from information from a number of the tutors. Some of the professions listed and open for applications were not known to the students, thus the role of the mentors was very important. Touwa had filled his application for a place in a University to learn Engineering. All the choices were the branches of Engineering like mechanical, civil and chemical. Mr Marijani noted that poor application and called Touwa for discussion. Touwa was asked to describe what the professions on a list provided. Apart from medicine, Touwa failed to show an understanding of what he was aspiring to do. Mr Marijani asked Touwa what Pharmacy was. Touwa was almost confident by answering that it was farming science like agriculture and that he did not want to do farming again as he had done enough in the village. Mr Marijani laughed and he then realised the poor level of understanding of the professions, and that was not only Touwa's problem but probably that of the whole sixth form class. He did not tell Touwa whether he was right or wrong but asked him to go to search in the books what that profession means in detail and to report the next morning. Touwa read the encyclopaedia that explained what the Pharmacy profession was and was utterly ashamed of the answer he had given to the Headmaster. In the morning all sixth form class were given a list of professions to search in the library, to understand all the listed trades before filling the application forms. Touwa went to see Mr Marijani and apologised for his ignorance, asked for a new application form and made first choice as Pharmacy. As he read for his A-level exams he sometimes wondered what he would look like as a Pharmacist as he had never seen a Pharmacist at work or someone who was a Pharmacist. He accepted the wisdom of Mr Marijani and decided to study for that profession, in the event he was selected to do Pharmacy. In additions to worries over examinations, students had lots of other worries, the exam results, the effect on the future and financial worries as dependence on mum or dad was not an option. After 14 years in school, many parents who were not that educated, were expecting some help. Many students had to opt for paid job due to such pressures.

Joining the newly created National Service which was a must after A-levels, was a serious worry as students could be drafted to fight in conflict zones. After the exams, the holidays followed, when Touwa worked before he joined National Service in January to June. Touwa made a weeks visit to his relatives at Nanjara to discover with glee that his younger brother, Ndesumbuka, had left home to join Olkejuado Secondary school, which was a boarding school. The second surprise was that Salema's new family was still growing. There was then Mamnana (a girl), Rosalia (a girl), Ndamejoi (a boy), Mangudo (a girl)Makinava (a girl)Edita (a girl), and Tete (a boy). Touwa was able to meet all the brothers and sisters as granddad welcomed Touwa in his celebratory fashion that involved a drink of '*mbege*' and a slaughtering of a lamb. The small family party helped to improve the kinship and improving the elders' bond. Touwa's uncle, Kimwai trimmed his hair proper in accordance to the services guidelines. Touwa, then an adult left for Ruvu National Service Camp. The theory and ideals of national service were good. The service achieved in building trust and friendship for people from all areas of the country, and with a military discipline and training instilled skills like house building, irrigation systems, road repair, farming, landscaping and the ideals of self reliant. After three months servicemen were moved to different camps to increase contacts and to enhance their specialized skills. Touwa was moved to Arusha camp to complete the remaining three months where they specialized in dairy farming. It was from that camp that all the sixth formers received results and placements. The newspaper copies that had the results were hot property as they were sold within five minutes of receipt. That first release was for A-level results arranged by schools. Each day, the week that followed, placements were declared. Touwa saw his selection for Nairobi University to become an engineer and he rejoiced as it was what he had chosen although not as a first choice. It was not long that a friend called by reading names of people selected to do courses that were not available in East Africa. Touwa's name appeared under Pharmacy to be studied at a place called Aston University in Birmingham in England. With two choices Touwa did not know how to celebrate but he did anyway, while waiting for confirmation from the education ministry. Before a letter from the ministry arrived, Salema received a letter from England, he knew it was for his son Touwa, as he could not read, he asked the younger brother to read. When he was told it was an acceptance letter to a University in England, Salema accompanied by Kimwai, his younger brother, friend and confidant, boarded a bus towards the Arusha camp to deliver the news personally to his son. The camp commander was also happy he allowed Touwa to leave the camp as only a few days were left to completion and that there were many steps needed for someone to leave the country like passports visas, finding birth certificates or evidence of birth at the home place, medicals, and numerous forms and documents to work on. With all those obstacles to climb, Touwa did not tell anyone that he was going abroad even to those who had read the newspaper, he denied having received confirmation. Touwa secured a teaching job at Kilimanjaro Boys secondary school a fee paying private school. It was at that school that he received a letter calling him to go to Dar es Salaam, the Capital city to make passport arrangements in order to proceed to England for his university education. His resignation from his job was a sad occasion for his students who had admired him and the staff who liked him. He made a trip to Nanjara to say bye to his sister Mkaleso, grandma, grandpa, father, uncles, brothers and sisters. Kimwai and Salema accompanied Touwa to Moshi town and said bye again as he left for Dar es Salaam, a city he was facing for the first time. Touwa with others who were going abroad were given accommodation for two week to enable the processing of passports and visas for travel to England.

CHAPTER 5

Away from the Country

The first flight:

The officials at the ministry of education handled the travelling arrangements efficiently. It started with knowledge on how to obtain the passport, the detailed steps of the process, like the photographs needed, the documents required, and where to go to get more advice or help. They planned and arranged the student's accommodation in Dar es Salaam, transport to the airport, getting flight tickets, and visas and eventually facilitated the flight away from the country. Arrangements had been put in place while the students were away in England, for monthly allowances to be paid to enable their upkeep like accommodation, food and social life. It was inside the East African Airways plane that some students started to put names they had read in newspapers to individuals. It was at that time; the students going to same University met and introduced themselves to one another. That was when Touwa met Mpina and Meriki who were going to Aston University for Pharmacy and Electronics respectively. The plane landed at Rome airport. That was significant as many who were Christians associated Rome with the home for the Pope the head of their religion, but no one on transit was allowed out of the plane as it was a very short stop. The only scare in flying till then was the turbulence experienced as the plane was flying over the Mediterranean Sea when drinks could fall from the tray used as a table. Many hearts were pumping faster than usual as all the students were awake. No one could sleep due to the high level of excitement due to the anticipation of going to new lands that they had read in geography books. On arrival, the students were received by an official from the British council who gave instructions on how to go to the city of London from Heathrow airport and how navigate to reach a bed and breakfast accommodation before to proceeding to designated Universities in all parts of the United Kingdom. The following day the students parted to their allocated schools. For some it was the first and last time they saw one another. Touwa, Mpina and Meriki took the train as instructed to Birmingham. It was when the three boys were in the train on the way to Birmingham that they noticed to their amazement that the train was faster than the cars. They had left a country with slow steam trains that had maximum speeds of 25 km per hour to see within a couple of days, a diesel or electric train travelling at 75 km per hour. That was amazing.

The University of Aston in Birmingham:

On arrival at Birmingham New street station, as instructed the boys took a taxi to Gosta Green, the main building of the University of Aston in Birmingham as it was known. The taxi took a while and charged a larger sum than the average. It was realised later that Gosta Green the University campus was very close to the train station. The taxi placed the new comers at the front door of the main building of the University of Aston in Birmingham. It was October; student registration and induction processes were completed earlier in September. The three new students were late but could not be returned home which was 6000 km away, so there was reception service delayed to receive overseas students who were late due to various complex travelling arrangements. The completion of registration that Friday, included a photo ID, instructions on where to find all facilities, guidance on shops, location of lecture rooms and the outline of the university departments with a key to an assigned room in the student residences. The three late but lucky new comers were to prepare for lessons which were to start on Monday, in two days' time. Touwa got a room on the 15th floor of a 24 floor tower called Lawrence tower. It was the first time Touwa had gone that high up in a building let alone to sleep in it. The extreme tiredness, the relaxation that he had arrived and the sheer happiness that he had seen Aston University, 6000km away from home, was enough to give him a sound sleep till the next morning. The next day Saturday was the only working day to go round the campus to see the lecture theatres, laboratories, student union, restaurants and shops. It was during those walkabouts that the three friends saw some other dark skinned people who were very few around the university campus. It was a shock to see people passing one another without saying 'hullo' or any kind of greetings and even refusing to reply if saluted for example, if one says 'good morning'. It was also a shock when a dark skinned man saluted decided to respond by starting a conversation with the three students. He was keen to know who they were and where they came from. He was speaking in English, but the three new students did not understand a word of what he said. It was a culture shock as the new comers started to have a hint of the many things that the new country they had visited would reveal. The curiosity of the new land just visited continued to be a surprise. The first worry was whether the anticipated first lecture that was only in a day's time on the Monday would be understood. Touwa woke up early that Monday morning, eager but worried whether he would understand the lecturers as he did not understand the first person he encountered. At nine o'clock prompt, the lecturer entered the hall and started speaking, Touwa was so happy to understand the whole lecture and every word used. Mpina, his classmate, also understood the lecture. In the class of 84 students, Touwa and Mpina were the only two dark skinned students. After the first lecture their confidence was high because of the near perfect understanding of their lecturer. That first lecture was an introduction to the range of subjects the students had to study in their quest to acquire a professional degree of Pharmacy. All the 84 students had good passes in A-level and were proud and confident that they were intellectuals but after that first lecture all that pride was reduced to being humble on the realisation of how little they knew even on the subjects already covered in high school. None of the students had heard, just to mention a few, subjects like *Pharmacology, Microbiology, Pharmacognosy, Physical chemistry, Medicinal chemistry, Pharmaceutics, Formulation, dispensing and Pharmaceutical Chemistry.*

Life at Aston was slowly becoming the well rehearsed routine of lectures, studying, reading, library time on weekdays and socializing by pub visits and some drinking on weekends. Touwa's new friend Dick was a local English boy who found it very amusing how Touwa could put a pencil that stayed held in place in his hair and that Dick could not do that. It was when Touwa allowed him to touch his hair to find a different texture and firmness that Dick understood how it was possible to hold a pencil in the hair. Dick and Touwa's friendship blossomed so well that

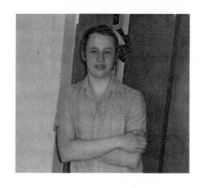

Touwas friend dick

they were known as friends by all classmates, lecturers and in social circles. The acquisition of more friends (pictured are Leone, Nahida with Touwa)was a factor in the reduction of Touwa's loneliness, but at times he remembered home.

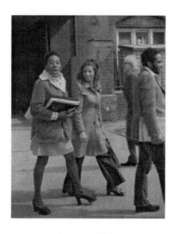

At aston Uni

Contact with home was difficult as communication systems were poor. Salema, Touwa's father would have to travel 70 km to access a phone, in contrast to Touwa who had a phone at his residence. The additional prohibitive cost of making an international call made it impossible to contact anyone at home in an emergency. Letter writing was an option but it took a month or two to get a reply. Receiving a letter from home was a moment of great pleasure. Writing letters was also a moment of pleasure due to the anticipated happiness of receiving a reply. Touwa's cousin, Lazaro, and his brother Ndesumbuka became a bridge through letter writing to convey to Touwa matters of interest about his family and friends. It was through such letters that Ndesumbuka who was then in Olkejuado Secondary school, revealed to Touwa how worried their father was every time he saw a plane flying over because it looked too small for his son to fit in. Salema was happy and reassured some years later, when he saw a plane that had landed to be bigger than the largest buses he had ever seen.

A University student:

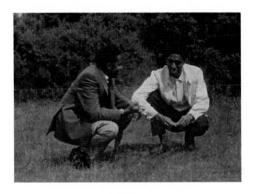

Meriki and Touwa at aston

117

Life as a student at the university was a privilege, rewarded with financial help, great aspirations, great freedom and the opportunity to make life long friends. The gaining of new knowledge, practical and theoretical with the possibility of teaching, or serving the government or community fuelled the need to work hard to achieve success. It was after the first term, a three month period that the students unanimously decided to question the Professor why they were not doing lessons that had relevance to Pharmacy. The students' lack of understanding was made clear by the Professor who replied by asking the students to ask him the same question at the end of the year. That question was never asked again because the second and third terms were used to cover the new subjects, the interrelation to Medicine and the provision of medicinal products for human and animal use. The originally portrayed character of pride and ignorance had worn off giving rise to humility and purpose of learning with the aspiration to become Pharmacists, aware of the amount of work needed to be done to reach the desired goal. The year end examinations were a source of worry and anxiety to all students. For overseas student however, failure could mean returning home without qualifications, a perceived shameful state of affairs that was dreaded by all. After the exams, there was a tense period waiting for results. The examination results were a reason to celebrate because all the three friends passed to proceed to year two. Touwa however did pass with an award in Chemistry, for which he was given a cash prize. He used that cash well by sharing with his brothers Ndesumbuka and Tabu who were also far away from home, had a drink with his friends Mpina, Dick and Meriki and above all bought a radiogram for his personal music enjoyment.

The second year was welcome with confidence due to improved social activities and ability to make more friends from many parts of the world. Touwa had friends from England, China, India, Iraq, Iran, Ireland, West Indies, Ghana, Sierra Leone, Nigeria, Kenya, Zimbabwe and Malawi. A compatriot, a girl called Macha (pictured with Mpina)joined Aston as a first year student in Pharmacy. The company of Leon (from the West Indies)and Nahida, a post graduate from Iraq, made the circle of friends greatly increased. With friends from so many countries the lonely moments of home sickness were greatly reduced. The confidence helped the students to get to know the Birmingham people better, giving the opportunity to get out more. It was during such socializing events that meeting with girls other than classmates occurred, leading to friendships. In time many of year two undergraduates acquired girl friends. Life styles shifted from simplicity to rather busy lifestyles. The new schedules included a complex array of promises or broken promises, dates, going to parties, cooking, shopping and drinking.

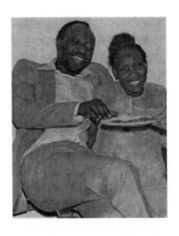

Mpina and Macha at Aston

The second year of study was an experiment that only course work would enable a student to pass. It was therefore to work hard during the whole year not near exam periods only as each home work counted as part of the final exam

119

in addition to submitting an essay as assigned by the course tutor. The social and academic changes affected many students. Some thought that the absence of exams meant an easy year, giving way to a relaxed way of life in regard to studies. That relaxation in the second year had profound effect on the progress of many students, as level of failures or repeats in the second year was above the previous year. For a pass to be granted in year two, a student had to have all the home wok submitted and certified passed, then the presentation of a written essay and an interview to explain the relevance of the written essay. For Touwa, it was his explanation and comment on the dangers that potent and dangerous hallucinogens could be made from simple medicinal molecules; that pleased Professor Wibberley who awarded a pass. With that pass Touwa started to see the goal of being a Pharmacist drawing closer to a possibility. Touwa also took the advice of searching for a summer job. He acquired a shop assistants work at Boots the Chemists, in a small shop in the Bull Ring Shopping centre in Birmingham. With that cash he sent small gifts or some cash to his brothers Ndesumbuka and Tabu who were in school and to his dad, a jacket or a blanket to help in keeping him warm.

Touwa's holiday, after the completion of year two was full of happy moments like getting a summer job and the meeting of a slim, pretty, dark skinned girl named Dorisi who became his girlfriend. It was at a christening party, at a house in St. Alban's road in Moseley in Birmingham when Dorisi and Touwa met. Dorisi, who had a smile that complemented her beauty, was a nurse who was studying to be a midwife. That new friendship changed Touwa, like his friends in similar circumstances, became conscious of his looks and acquired fashion dressing. In short he became smarter. That busy summer holiday appeared short as the time for the final, year three, was fast approaching. The lectures for year three undergraduates started. Thoughts of what that year would throw at the students were of great concern, reducing that happy cheerful holiday mood to a sombre, serious, thoughtful and reflective period.

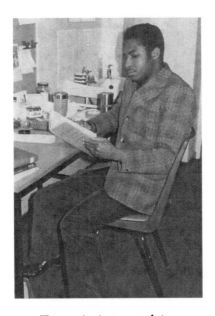

Touwa At Aston studying

The year was hard because more and newer subjects were introduced, coupled with practical work that mimic the reality in the field of Pharmacy, like dispensing and making of various pharmaceutical formulations. Examples were creams, ointments, eye or ear drops and suspensions. The science subjects learned were meant to prepare pharmacists to work in areas of making medicinally active chemicals, formulating such products to usable medicines, ensuring correct dosage, preparing the medicine in a form easy to administer like a tablet or syrup, then packaged and labelled properly. Finally the product could be presented to the public with guidance on the proper usage. In addition, Pharmacists were also chemists that could work in chemical analysis, toxicology and testing for quality and purity in the chemical industry. Furthermore, Pharmacists were trained in bacterial and viruses' treatment and resistance awareness and problem solving. To ensure awareness of future developments, an introduction to new and emerging therapies like radioactivity and gene therapy in medicine was discussed with the future influence of computers. Many of the overseas students had the phobia of failure to return home with no qualifications. That worry forced a change in behaviour like a significant reduction in social activity in weekdays to a day per week and in a weekend. Touwa, Dick, Lam and Hirji shared ideas and study moments as they had developed friendships during the second year. The study meetings, library visits, writing of experimental work, attending study meetings with group tutor and writing or correcting reports dominated life in that third year. The approach of the examinations time was also when students needed support from family and friends. As all Touwa's friends were in the same situation of the need for support, the only option was to give each other comforting words when assuming a poor outcome in the results. Some girl friends who understood the pressure of exams gave some support, but some pressed and insisted on carrying on socially as usual. Touwa's girlfriend, Dorisi, had just done her exams and passed; hence she understood the situation and gave the best support a man could get.

On the first day of the examinations that lasted for a period of two weeks all the students were advised to eat light meals and drink in moderation and to arrive early in order to be relaxed ready for entry into the Great Hall, that had a seating of a thousand students from many departments, to be assigned a seat. All Pharmacy students were on time but a small group of 'Combined Honours' degree students who were rushing, overfilled a lift which jammed and stopped on its way down in Lawrence tower! It was by sheer luck that an engineer was visiting, who was able to release them. That group of students arrived at the Great Hall just as the papers were being handed to the students. That last minute distraction eased the exam tension as one could imagine the tension of those who came late. The tensest period in life for Touwa and his close friends was during the time of writing examination that spun for two weeks. That was followed by an equally worrying period of a month before the time for results. During that waiting time most local students had left for home leaving Lawrence tower a ghost building with very few overseas students. To add to their worry, the overseas students had to move to a smaller building in order to use the tower for conference guests. After the results all were to vacate all University accommodations.

Touwa had secured a position of training as a Pre-registration student at Dudley Road Hospital pending the outcome of results. Touwa had not lived outside Lawrence tower for the three years, so he had no idea of the type and cost of accommodation, unlike his friends Mpina and Meriki who had lived outside the campus for a period. One clear fact was that after the declaration of results, the University did not take any more responsibility to graduates accommodation. It was then time to vacate the premises and say good bye to Aston University. The results would determine the mood of the good byes. It was during a casual talk between Touwa and Dorisi, his girlfriend that the subject of accommodation arose. Touwa did not want to show how he knew nothing of life outside the campus. Dorisi suggested contacting her friend who was completing her studies and would vacate a flat at Salisbury road in Moseley. It was good news that the flat would be vacant and further more the landlord accepted the occupancy by Touwa and Dorisi. Touwa had then no more problems only the wait for the results. It was a Thursday when many students woke up nervously, because it was the day for results. Those local students who had gone home returned to see their results that were posted on the main notice board. Touwa and Mpina walked slowly without talking to the main building while Meriki went to the Engineering building where his results were posted. All the 84 Pharmacy students including all others from a number of departments for biological sciences were around the notice board. Everyone wanted to see the results quick, some left fast but some were reading to see who was above or below them. It was therefore a push and be pushed atmosphere. Mpina, who was taller than Touwa, was expected to read both results. As soon as Mpina reached a distance he could read, he made the names and shouted loudly to Touwa: *"You have passed, your name and mine are here."* Those words were said by many taller friends who were acting for shorter colleagues and for some of the girls. There were four grades of passes but initially the grade was not important. Before Touwa could see his name, he trusted Mpina and started to rejoice telling each other "congratulations". All the students passed except five who had to complete one paper to pass for the degree. After shouting, congratulating each other, shaking hands, patting others backs, hugging and kissing that went on for a period, it was time for the few who could not read the results at first got a chance to read the detail and find their grades.

There were four grades: First, Upper second, Lower second, Third and Pass. Touwa and Mpina ware in division 'Upper Second'. It was a good pass because there were four passes as first division, eight passed in upper second division, twenty five passes in lower second, thirty eight in third division, six were pass level and there were three who had to repeat a subject and eventually passed to gain a degree called Bachelor of Science in Pharmacy(BSc. Pharmacy.)It was that degree which enabled the entry to training termed 'pre registration' for a year before one is granted a licence to practice independently as a Pharmacist.

That day, the day of the results was a day to celebrate. The largest and most raucous group was at Aston Student Union, where there was music dancing drinking. At about midnight, a new craze was invented: It was *'streaking'*. How that craze started was not quite clear because drinks had started clouding judgements. Reliable sources reported that a girl called a bluff to a boy that if he dared to take all his clothes and run in the street to his flat then he would qualify to be her boy friend. It is amazing what fun a drink can bring. The boy showed his love by striping to the last piece of cloth and ran from the student union to Lawrence tower through a public street followed by his girlfriend who was carrying his clothes accompanied by many spectators. When they returned to the student Union to enjoy the new hero status for those who dared, news of the craze became a public matter, copy cat 'streaking' became the enjoyment of the night as more, and more girls encouraged their boys to streak. Some did not need encouragement, making the path between the student union and Lawrence tower a spectre for 'streaking'. The next morning it was the day of packing belongings to go home or to other lodgings outside the campus. It was a sad day for so many good byes but also a joyful day of achievement. All the graduates, classmates and friends knew that good bye was temporary as they would meet on graduation day, after that occasion they probably would never see one another again.

The graduation was the most colourful ceremony any University performs. The graduation ceremony at Aston was grand. The Chancellor was conferring degrees to more that one thousand graduates. It started with the post graduate degrees of Doctorates of Science and Philosophy, follower by Masters of Science or Arts then finally the Bachelor degrees. The local students had parents with them who took pictures, laughed, chatted and even went for meals. For Touwa and his overseas friends it was a lonely time that reminded them of home and parents. The three year absence from home and family had matured the overseas students that they arranged their own celebration with friends they had acquired during the period at Aston. At Graduation Touwa was accompanied by Dorisi, his girlfriend. Mpina and Meriki were similarly accompanied. The talk had then focussed on work and future employment, as at each stage of life the uncertainty of the future ferments a little worry even for successful graduates like Touwa, Mpina and Meriki. The three graduates were all aware that the days of receiving stipends were over and money had to be earned through work. It was the beginning of thinking like a working man.

CHAPTER 6

Transition period

New life style:

It was without much difficulty to pack the few belongings from the student room at Lawrence tower on the Aston campus to a flat at Salisbury road. It was a new type of life with new responsibilities that Touwa never thought of before. The payment of gas, water, electricity, council tax and rent bills were the initial shock of the real working life. Budgeting for travelling expenses working clothes that had to show a higher level of smartness were other new issues. It took time for the newly qualified Pharmacist to understand and comprehend the basic life essentials unlike the life he led for the past 17 years of student life. Dorisi, who had a better understanding of how things were done, slowly stirred Touwa in the right direction to the understanding and comprehension. It was a slow process that eventually became easy. Touwa's work as a pre-registration student was a paid job, enabling him and Dorisi who also worked, to start a life with a good financial standing. With time, Touwa's working routine was becoming the norm, and the regular shopping for food, the cooking, washing, keeping the flat tidy, and learning to live with a room mate was slowly getting to be understood. Life was turning to a new normality, but with drastically new and complex responsibilities. Touwa started to have a different attitude in life, changing from a student to a worker. That new outlook of life started with the realisation of proper dressing up at work and in social occasions, issues of money, savings, wealth creation including the care of loved ones and the future thinking of what the career in Pharmacy would offer. The routine of work that was then normal to Touwa came to a stop, the day a letter was received from the Ministry of Health in Dar es Salaam. The letter from Dar es Salaam simply gave orders to return home to complete the pre registration locally and that refusal would be a breach of the terms for the scholarship. Touwa as well as Mpina, who was also working decided to accept the order and prepare to head for home, Tanzania. It was in a sombre mood and sadness that Touwa broke the leaving news to his dear girl friend, Dorisi. It was a shock to Doris who had grown fond of Touwa and had developed to love him very much. It was then they realised they loved one another intensely and none wanted the separation. The feelings were mutual, Touwa was thinking with no easy answer while Dorisi was also thinking with no obvious solution.

It was in the evening when they were eating a good dinner that Dorisi had prepared that they talked candidly on the subject of Touwa's plan to go home. Doris did not eat much but she was sobbing and crying with intensity that continued to bed time. Touwa tried to console Dorisi as the cries went on for a long time. With lots of *'I love you'* with kisses, the sobbing subsided and logical thinking could then be possible. In the morning as Touwa was running to catch the bus on the way to work, when he asked Dorisi a question: *'Will you go with me to Africa?'* But before Dorisi could utter a word Touwa was in the bus that had sped away. At work Touwa was pondering on the significance of the question and he was preparing himself for either a *'Yes or No'.* Touwa finished work, arrived at his flat before Dorisi. He had neither flowers nor a little present to give to Dorisi for possibility of changing a *'no'* to a *'yes'.* When Dorisi arrived, Touwa remembered the tradition at home that made people happy. It was food and a drink. He asked Dorisi if she fancied going to a restaurant. A walking distance away in Moseley village at a nice cafe, they had a meal and an opportunity to talk. That was when the question was answered. Dorisi and Touwa had known one another for just over a year but had only lived together in a flat for two months. When the answer was *'yes'* Dorisi and Touwa talked of the future in a candid and grown up manner. It was agreed that Touwa would go first to arrange for job and accommodation and Dorisi to follow in a month's time. With that note, they finished their meal, went to the flat thinking and talking about the planned future. There were a few nights of laughter, talking and happiness as Touwa packed his belongings to leave England to head home and see his brothers and sisters whose numbers had increased since he left Africa. First were the seniors, Salema, Shenji, Yohana, Mamacholo, Alina and Mamoroi and a unique opportunity to know all the step brothers and sisters that were born when Touwa was away. The list of the children of Salema from the wives: Mkasu, Alina and Mamoroi are given below. (g—Symbolising girls*)*

Mkasu (late)Children:

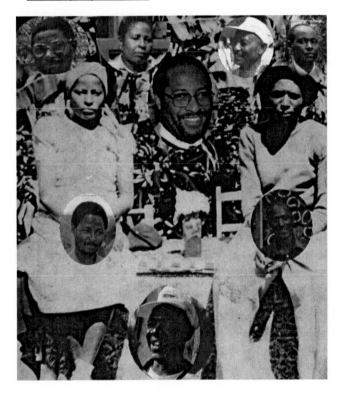

Chilren of Mkasu with Salema

1-Salimu,
2-Mkaleso (g),
3-Touwa,
4-Ndesumbuka,
5-Melikoi,
6-Tabu,
7-Tabuni (*Kimbulumbulu*)
8-Mashaka (*adopted*)

Alina's children:

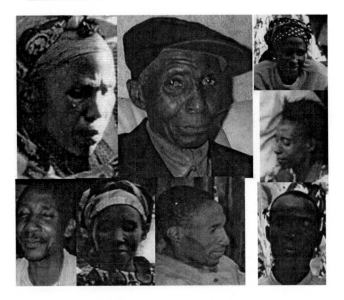

Children of alina with Salema

9-Mkabasia, (g)
10-Yonaa,
11-Mamkwe (g)
12-Mkwe,
13-Mshiki (g)
14-Mkosi

Mamoroi's Children:

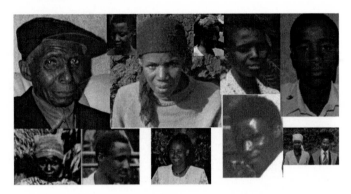

Children of Mamoroi with Salema

15-Mamnana (g),
16-Fortunata (g),
17-Rosa, (g)
18-Ndamejoi,
19-Edita, (g)
20-Tete,
21-Makinavei (g)
22-Nakuvesia *(Kinyeti)*

It was also Touwa's desire, he thought, to see and talk to all the neighbours and school friends like Failosi, Shirima, Lazaro, Arobo, Modesta, Rita, Mwandafu, Kamasho, Kalisti, Jenofefa, Krispini, Albina, Lusia, Redemta, and Silayo. The beloved uncle Kimwai would possibly wait eagerly to see and hear a lot from Touwa. The neighbours too, were interested to hear stories of Touwa's travels. Touwa was mentally prepared to tell the sequence of events that he experienced over the period he was away, stressing the achievements, like his degree qualification and what it was called, including the work he then could do.

That thought of his family was a reminder of the poverty that was left behind him as he travelled away from the village. He spent most of the money buying presents like shirts, jumpers, and a blanket for his grandfather. He tried to get little things to ensure that all close family members got something. He was also given in addition to travel ticket, a shipping pro-forma invoice for the government to pay the shipping charges. He packed a trunk with books and anything he owned for shipment. Although Touwa had always found it easy to leave and go, that leaving episode was the most difficult as he was in love. Before he boarded the train to London and eventually to Heathrow airport, he asked Dorisi to keep her promise, and with a passionate kiss he went fast to the platform to board the train.

The proud graduates:

In the train, Touwa and Mpina talked all the way on family, soon to see, work, and girls, those that were left behind before and after Aston University. The East African Airways plane that took the two boys to Aston University was the same plane that was returning them home, as, graduates and professional young men who were probably confident and conceited. The other graduates that met in the plane equally expressed pride and high opinion of their newly acquired graduate status. The talk was mainly on the level of degree attained and the profession they achieved, the salary and the position of work in the organisations they aspired to join. The way some graduates spoke could give the impression that Tanzania would change drastically on their arrival. The numerous tales of experience in the new country, generated great moments of laughter, making the overnight flying pass quickly such that the landings and take offs at Rome and Nairobi on the way to Dar es Salaam were barely noticed. The humid and hot air was a shock, possibly one of many, that the arrival at Dar es Salaam met the graduates. They had three years of lower temperatures; they had to acclimatise to that new weather. The profuse sweating made their brilliantly white shirts stick to their bodies, a phenomenon they had forgotten. Some had forgotten how to be fluent in Swahili, the national language, it was sometimes embarrassing, but worse was to come as many graduates had forgotten their local dialect, when they met parents or other relatives as it was not spoken for three years. Those who had really forgotten were marked as uneducated by their family, a comment that set them down a peg or two in their self acclaimed importance. Touwa and Mpina did not experience any problems in the language switch because they had kept each other company for three years both socially and in lectures. The checks done by custom officers were less rigorous to students who were returning home, so Touwa had a speedy exit to meet Kimwai, his uncle, who came to Dar es Salaam airport. Touwa understood but could not talk fluently in Kichagga at first but during the 650 km journey to Nanjara, Touwa listened to Kimwai telling all that had happened during the three years that Touwa was away. When the bus was close to home, Touwa heard a lot of people speaking the dialect, that triggered his memory of the days he was in Nanjara and the dialect fluency returned.

The folks of Nanjara:

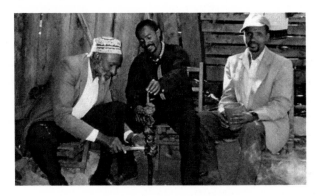

Meat eating and drinking

When he met his father and all the relatives, he greeted them in the dialect and he was respected for remembering after three years. There were some folk who knew few words of English. They decided to test Touwa whether he really was in England. Touwa replied their question in fluent, fast spoken language that they could not understand, so they changed the conversation to the dialect. The mutual respect was established and Salema hoisted a party of 'mbege' drinking, meat eating (pictures are cousin Mtele, *(sharing the meat)*Tabuni and uncle Sumaili)and singing the old songs that continued to the night reminding Touwa that he was back home. One local teacher, Kamasho, an uncle to Touwa's best school friend, Shirima, gave a loan to Touwa. It was a scooter to ride and travel more efficiently to visit friends. That good gesture of lending the scooter to Touwa was supported by Kimwai, Touwa's uncle, who supervised and ensured safety in the use of the equipment. Kamasho, the teacher, was happy that there was a learned person in the village. Touwa used the two weeks of holiday, talking to the village folk, school pupils and students from colleges about his overseas experience. He probably was one of the first few in Nanjara to attain that level of high education and the first one as a Pharmacist. That knowledge made him humble and approachable unlike some who were so arrogant that they did not return to the village to see their parents. The two week holiday appeared to end fast due to the many commitments of Touwa. He visited all his friends, but for those who were not in the village, Touwa went to visit their parents. The closest school friend, Shirima, was then working away from the village so Touwa could only talk to his parents. The other close friend Lazaro was working in the local town, so Touwa arranged to meet with him on the way to Dar es Salaam. It was the day he was leaving for Dar es Salaam to start his Pharmacy work training at Muhimbili Hospital that Touwa went to see his father to tell him of Dorisi, the girl he left in UK. Salema's eyes were wide opened with happiness when Touwa showed the picture. Salema's happy expression encouraged Touwa to confirm the expected visit of Dorisi and the possibility of a wedding. Before Salema could say a word, Touwa said goodbye, got on his scooter, and sped way promising his dad more detailed information in a letter.

At Muhimbili:

At Moshi town, Touwa and his friend Lazaro met. Their meeting was a happy moment of mixed emotions and fond memories and played a role in cementing their friendship that was close, amicable and deemed to continue for a long time. On his journey to Dar es Salaam, Touwa reflected on his life and focused on the future which appeared complicated. He thought of work, pay, money, self support, parent support, brother and sister's support, accommodation, wife and eventually kids. With never ending thoughts like those, Touwa drifted to sleep as the coach was speeding towards Dar es Salaam. On waking up Touwa was at Kariakoo in Dar es Salaam where he had to alight. He was to report to Muhimbili hospital but he did not know where it was. Touwa knew two places in Dar es Salaam, the Ministry of Education and that his cousin Mtele lived in the city. He did not know how to go to any of those places, as he knew less of Dar es Salaam than Birmingham. He asked a man the directions to Muhimbili. The man suggested a taxi as he was a taxi driver. The drive to Muhimbili took a while as the driver used scenic routes pretending to show the city as he realised Touwa did not know Dar es Salaam. On arrival at Muhimbili, he paid the hefty fare, just as he did in Birmingham, for journeys that he could just walk. Touwa was expected at Muhimbili. He was given a one room accommodation and told to report to the Senior Pharmacist to start the training.

Muhimbili was a large national hospital that was also a teaching centre for Medical doctors, nurses, health inspectors, Midwives, laboratory and Pharmacy technicians. It was a place to meet many people, especially colleagues as the hospital was a training centre for Medical, Dental and Pharmacy pre registration trainees. Touwa met Mpina again, including another new Pharmacy trainee, Mapunda. There were in addition, Medical trainees like Mlele, Kangethe, Mroso and Mkunde who became friends of Touwa. The relaxed atmosphere at Muhimbili hospital was in stark contrast to life at a UK hospital that was manifested by time, schedules, deadlines and inspections. At Muhimbili the pace of work was slow, but at the pharmacy, the input of new students namely Mapunda, Touwa and Mpina, saw a faster pace of work, better preparations of medicines, supply of smoother creams and ointments and better teaching of the technicians. The senior pharmacist was happy at the work quality and ethics including the changes done to the pharmacy on medicines arrangement for easier access, the introduction of checks and accountability including setting up of departments within the pharmacy to augment efficiency. The quality of changes that were introduced by the new trainees was noticed by patients and the senior doctors. That initial impact attracted requests to teach nurses and pharmacy technicians, duties that were carried out diligently. The work at Muhimbili was not heavy but Touwa had a lot in his mind, the expected visit of his girlfriend, Dorisi, with the view for a marriage, wedding ceremony, and the anticipated travel to visit the parents with the view to get a good house to live. Despite all these thoughts, Touwa had to accompany Kangethe and Mpina for the regular visits to the pub for a drink. Those visits enabled Touwa to know the Dar es Salaam city. Cousin Mtele was living at a two bedroom flat at a busy road junction at Kariakoo in Dar es Salaam. It was sometimes very noisy from the large trucks that moved goods from the port of Dar es Salaam to the land locked countries of Zambia, Rwanda and Burundi, even to countries as far as Zimbabwe. Touwa and Mtele met often, as that was the only family contact he had in Dar es Salaam. It was not long before Touwa told Mtele all his future plans including the arrival of Dorisi. Mtele became concerned when Touwa indicated his worry on matters of accommodation. Touwa's fears were reduced when Mtele assured Touwa that he would help.

The arrival of Dorisi:

Touwa showed Mtele the letter, from Dorisi, an airmail letter which had to be opened carefully as the written piece of blue paper that formed the letter was cleverly folded to act as an envelope, thus reducing weight and postage cost. In that letter she confirmed the arrival date. That date which had to be remembered was Sunday the 15th December 1974. Touwa had to plan the meeting and transport from the airport to collect his beloved Dorisi. Life at Muhimbili was with Dorisi in mind, as work was becoming a routine of dispensing and making creams and ointments or lotions.

Early on the arrival date Touwa accompanied by Mpina, boarded the airport bus to collect their guest scheduled to arrive at 10.00 a.m. by Egypt air. At the airport the two Aston graduates checked the arrival timetable and were happy to see the plane flight number and arrival time as per travel itinerary. At 10.00 a.m. the two friends who were at the balcony where one could see landings and taxing, expected to see the huge Boeing 747 Egypt air coming for landing, but up to 10.30 am there was no plane. Mpina, in his usual charismatic manner, suggested that the delay may be a hint that she made a bluff and she was not coming. Touwa's confidence was wearing down a bit so he took the letter, double checked the date, the flight number and that it was Egypt air, to see the match with the arrival notice. At that second check, the word 'delayed' was written in the place of the arrival time. Touwa and Mpina sat silently pondering the differences in efficiency between the country they went for studies and their own. As Mpina observed Touwa drifting to sadness, he suggested going to drink a glass of beer, a suggestion that was warmly welcome. As the hours passed, the two fiends talked much about their life experiences before going to UK, while in UK and after their studies in Birmingham and at Muhimbili. After a snack at midday, the waiting continued until the elusive Egypt air would ever make a landing. It was about 3.30 pm when the arrivals board indicated 'arrival' time for the Egypt air instead of 'delayed' notice. It was at 4.00pm that a large plane was approaching the Dar es Salaam airport for landing and as it came closer it was Egypt air. The question that remained was whether Dorisi was in or not! The huge Boeing 747 approached the runway noisy but majestically, until the tyres touched the Dar e Salaam tarmac and dust. When the plane had stopped the doors were open to let the passengers out, and it was by luck that Mpina and Touwa could see clearly as the passengers walked down the stairs from the plane to the tarmac. The two friends scrutinised each passenger in a bid to identify Doris. Touwa was getting worried as more and more passengers came down with no sign of Dorisi. But wow! A young woman appeared. It was her, Dorisi, looking majestic, with an afro hair style, a white blouse, a dark skirt, just above the knee. On her shoulder, she hung a medium size hand bag and on her left hand she held her hand luggage. She stopped for a bit may be worried as it was the first time her feet would step on an African soil, or to search for the host, the boy she loved, so much as to travel 8000 km to be with. She came to fulfil a promise. At the bottom of the steps from the plane, she stepped on the hot tarmac and stopped again. That time she was so happy and smiled. Her teeth were brilliant white, visible clearly at a good distance. She heard her name called, she dropped her luggage and waved to Touwa and Mpina who were equally ecstatic. With her boyfriend around, Doris's confidence was elevated as she hurriedly proceeded to immigration to enter Tanzania. It was not long; Touwa and

Dorisi were re—united as agreed on the Tanzanian soil. The three months of separation had not diminished their love or their sense of humour. The journey to Muhimbili was on a taxi, the initial talk was on that plane delay and Mpina, and Touwa's waiting. It was revealed by Dorisi that the plane left UK on time, delayed in Cairo for six hours with extra unscheduled stops at Entebbe and Zanzibar. Mpina commented that Dorisi had in her first trip to Africa a lesson in that word 'delay'. With laughter Dorisi also commented that the huge trucks and cars on the roads reminded her of World War II films she used to see, meaning she had gone back in time. Mpina agreed and added that Tanzania may be a century behind and only running very fast could catch the others and that he could not see the relaxed Africans making an attempt to run fast. The arrival at Muhimbili coincided with dinner time, which was a welcome relief since everyone was then very tired. Dorisi and Touwa continued talking and introductions to friends until late when everyone went to sleep. The next day was work as usual, dispensing, teaching junior staff or at the school for pharmacy technicians. Life was then back to normal, except Touwa's thoughts to find a house, as he was then not alone. Touwa's friends like Mpina helped to advance Dorisi's knowledge of life in Tanzania, while the new friend, Kangethe, a medical intern, introduced her to the social life which was mainly drinking. His frequent travels to the city earned him the nick name 'Mr Stanley' the great African explorer. Dorisi was introduced to Mtele, Touwa's cousin who was living at Kariakoo in Dar es Salaam. It happened that Mtele was travelling to Nanjara that very week to see his family. Touwa took the opportunity to ask Mtele to see Salema to announce the arrival of Dorisi, as a gesture of respect to his father that Touwa was not living alone. With that small traditional act in place life was again at its normal slow pace.

Yohana at 80:

It was during that period of happiness, great social life, ample relaxation, that the beloved Yohana, Touwa's grandmother passed away. Touwa left Dorisi in the care of Mpina and Kangethe, to go to the grandmother's funeral. She had died peacefully in her sleep. Had Touwa gone to Nanjara, as soon as Dorisi arrived,

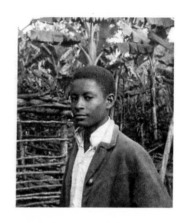

Ndesumbuka in Secondary school

Yohana, the beloved grandmother could have seen her grandson's future wife. Touwa's brother, Ndesumbuka was exceedingly sad because he had postponed a planned talk with Yohana, the talk that was never to happen, a point of long term sorrow and regret. When Ndesumbuka was going to Muhoho high school, Yohana called him for a chat but the boy was rushing to meet his mates, telling her that they would talk when he came back the following holiday, when Yohana commented that she may not be there. Taking that as a joke Ndesumbuka left for school. The death of Yohana aged 80, occurred before the return of Ndesumbuka. Touwa's younger brother. The week of stay at Nanjara, was the opportunity that Touwa took to talk to his father about the future plans of celebrations for the welcome for Dorisi. The plans were agreed amicably.

Dorisi early experiences in Africa:

On the way to Dar es salaam Touwa was planning a return journey to introduce Dorisi to the whole family. It had to be after the festive season of Christmas. Dorisi experienced her first Christmas in Africa. It was different and in contrast to UK, there was little of present giving or cards but close family members meet with friends at a house of one family member. The gathering involved, drinking, food eating consisting mainly of a slaughtered goat, chicken or goose, including music, dancing and lots of chatting. Many people however travelled to their ancestral homes to celebrate Christmas with their parents. Touwa however celebrated with his cousin Mtele and his family, as he could not secure another week or two away from work. After Christmas life was a little dull as too much was spent in celebrations making it necessary to wait till another pay day. It was well known that when that day arrived it was marked with the usual late night raucous chats that were heard at the interns mess by those returning from enjoying by spending their hard earned cash.

It was time, to travel with Dorisi to Nanjara to meet Shenji, the granddad, Salema the dad, the two wives of Salema, the brothers and sisters, the nephews and nieces, including the many friends of the family of Nanjara village. That was the time Touwa was nervous. A train journey was planned taken on a Friday morning, with the expectation of arriving Moshi on Saturday morning, proceeding to Nanjara to arrive between 4 and 6 pm. That was safer but

143

very slow in contrast to the fast couch travel that was prone to collisions. The slow train would take 25 hours from Dar es Salaam to Moshi town, stopping at all stations. At each station water and coal was replenished and more passengers came on board. At a steep climb the speed could be as low as 15 Km per hour. The train route passed through bush land and Dorisi was amazed to see no houses and very few huts, and sometimes wild life consisting of mainly monkeys. At one station called Mombo, the train developed a mechanical problem, delaying the travel for four hours. That delay meant that the arrival at Moshi town and the next journey to Nanjara could be in jeopardy as the couple were expected in the afternoon. At Moshi town, nearly 75 Km to Nanjara, there was the problem in getting a coach as it was late afternoon. The last coach that was leaving was full but Touwa and Dorisi got a standing position to start the second part of the journey. It was then 24 hours that had passed without proper sleep. That journey took five hours most of which was standing and arriving at Nanjara bus stop at eight in the night. The welcome party left for home at seven sensing that the last bus had arrived. At Nanjara it was pitch dark, Dorisi had never experienced such darkness; the only light was the stars in the sky. Touwa started to proceed to go in the direction of his home with Dorisi following closely as she hardly could see Touwa. It was also the first time Touwa was alone at night without a local guide. After a little walk Touwa stopped, he could not see the path. Dorisi's heart was pumping fast with fear. He asked Dorisi to go back to follow the larger path. Dorisi asked if Touwa was lost. Touwa admitted to miss his road but confident he would find the proper road. Dorisi was so frightened and shivering from cold and fear. She asked if there were lions that would eat them. That made Touwa worried and ashamed that he forgot his way home. The second route was clear and Touwa and Dorisi walked, past Touwa's old school, the dispensary and eventually saw a light. Touwa shouted to alert Dorisi that the light came from his auntie's house. Dorisi was relieved and walked fast towards that light. When Touwa said hello, the cousins came out with lanterns as they were expecting the arrival of Touwa and Dorisi. Dorisi was happy to meet Touwa's closest family. There was the added bonus of meeting two young girls who spoke some English. Dorisi gained her usual smile and with the help of the two twin cousins, Albina and Lusia, the walk for the last kilometre to Touwa's ancestral home was a relaxing and a happy one. The reception was not less triumphant, although it was at night, all brothers and sisters were still waiting, and a chicken meal was prepared. All present appreciated the tiredness of the journey and allowed the couple to go to sleep earlier than planned.

Dorisi first holiday at Nanjara:

Early in the morning the calling of Shenji was heard as he arrived to see Dorisi. He was not alone but accompanied by a number of neighbours who were keen to see a black person who was not African. When they were told her original country as St Kitts, many of the Nanjara had no knowledge of that land, for simplicity it was agreed she came from America. Salema was too excited to wait for a visit, so he travelled from his boundary farm to see his daughter in law to be. That visit made Shenji the granddad, start a party. He gave Touwa a sheep to slaughter, Touwa called Failosi to help and Failosi called Kimwai to assist. When that drama of who could slaughter that sheep continued, Dorisi was being entertained by a large number of admirers, sisters, cousins, neighbours and friends. Albina and Lusia the first cousins she met were always by her side to protect and as interpreters to make conversation possible. Doris was loved by all from Shenji, the grandfather, Salema, the dad, all brothers and sisters, including all Touwa's old school mates. The love, the admiration, the protection, the care and being the centre of attention made Doris relaxed and felt as if she was a Nanjara born girl. The sheep was eventually

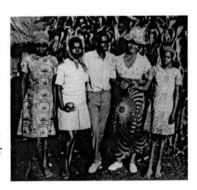

Doris at Nanjara

slaughtered, the meet roasted, the *'mbege'* shared with generosity and the guests arriving in droves, which was the start of an impromptu party for the welcome of Dorisi to Nanjara. The party ended with lots of singing with the view to meet at Salema's boundary farm the next day. It was there at Salema's boundary farm that a hint of the wedding plans was discussed. The holiday was a success. It was on the outbound journey to Dar es Salaam that Doris hinted on the love of the welcome she received at Nanjara.

CHAPTER 7

Work, Marriage, and Parenthood

The first flat and marriage:

The life at the intern's mess was getting boring especially when cash flow was low. It was very quiet with very few sports facilities. Dorisi was also fed up with the food at the interns mess. To avoid boredom and the staff mess food Touwa, and Dorisi, went to see cousin Mtele most evenings where they could cook a dish different from the mess usual. It was in one of such evenings that Mtele revealed to Touwa that he was leaving to go back to Mwadui Diamond mines to continue with his work. He added that Touwa could occupy the flat afterwards on the understanding that he took care of Mtele's household properties like his good quality settee and keep supporting his dependent bother that was in training. It was an offer that could not be refused as Dorisi liked the flat too. Touwa's major issues had then been reduced to just one. The four major issues that disturbed Touwa's head as he graduated were the plan and arrival of Dorisi in Dar es Salaam, the job, a flat and an eventual marriage. With happiness Touwa and Dorisi returned to their residential place at Muhimbili with plans on how to set their flat to their own image. It was during that happy moment they decided on the date of the marriage which was Saturday 15th March 1975. When Mtele was informed of the intended marriage and date, he approved and accepted taking major responsibility on behalf of his uncle Salema. Due to financial constraints travelling to Dar es Salaam by Touwa's family was not possible but a compromise was agreed that was to hold a small marriage ceremony in Dar es Salaam then at a later date, a family wedding at Nanjara. With that compromise, the small ceremony at Dar was planned. Time passed rather fast with the wedding preparations and work, that the 15th day of March became the tomorrow, when at ten o'clock, Dorisi and Touwa including two witnesses Mtele and Moshiro were at a registry office. It was a short brief process involving an exchange of vows and signing a register that made Dorisi and Touwa become legally married. The reception for the marriage celebration was on the third floor roof top of Mtele's flat that was at a busy junction between Msimbazi and Kariakoo streets in the Kariakoo district in Dar es Salaam. Although it was a small gathering, the happiness the warmth, the comradeship, the love, in addition to the food and drinks, made the small wedding ceremony into a huge occasion that was memorable and respectable. The drinking, eating, dancing and chatting was

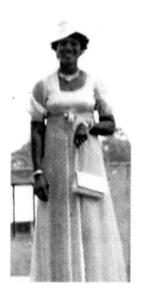

Dorisi at her wedding

concluded late in the night when Dorisi and Touwa, then Mr and Mrs returned to Muhimbili to plan for their next traditional marriage ceremony at Nanjara. Dorisi and Touwa were then man and wife but they had a marriage ceremony to complete following the Chagga traditions and in the presence of the parents, grandparents, other close family relatives and almost the whole of the folk of Nanjara village. That second ceremony was to take place a month after the first one. Salema started preparing the drinks and food for the celebration of the marriage of his third child, a second son. Touwa and Dorisi made preparations to go to Nanjara, that time they did not use the slow train but a coach that left Dar es Salaam for Moshi, and the connecting buses to Nanjara were according to the declared timetables. On arrival at Nanjara, there was a warm welcome.

The Salema compound was in the process of decoration with flowers, banana leaves and an evergreen shrub known as *'isale'*, a plant that was claimed to be nucleus of the Chagga people as it was believed that where an *'isale'* can flourish, a Chagga person can also make a home. Pioneers like Shenji who travelled to new lands were said to carry *'isale'* to plant near their hut. The plant was used as a border around the hut and very seldom used as fodder for animals. While those decorations were being put up, sweet voices of young girls practising their wedding chant could be heard. The next day, that was the day

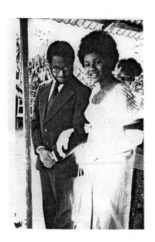

**Touwa and Dorisi
at Nanjara wedding**

for the wedding celebrations. It was tradition that the bride and groom start walking into Salema's compound, being showered with petals and lots of singing. At the reception after sitting down, *'mbege'* was served. During the early drinking period, the crowd was calm and speeches by friends of Touwa declaring him as a married man and offerings of advice were conducted. Wedding food was then goat meat roasted on a log fire and offered to the bride and groom. To signify their union Touwa was to cut a piece of meat to feed Dorisi who was to do likewise. It was after that mutual feeding, that the rest of the guests started eating and drinking in earnest. Music and dancing would have started when the older folk would leave the younger crowd with the bride and groom to feel free to dance and chat. The older folk sat around a burning log fire to keep warm, chat notably praising Salema for the achievement. With plenty to drink and eat, there was vigour and a raucous nature on the dance floor and a start of singing around the log fire. At a point it sounded as if it was a competition between the singing and the radiogram playing. When the chorus of *'haya, o haya haya hee'* was very loud one could tell it was a good party and that there was plenty to eat. The dancing was coming to an end due to darkness as one could not see one with whom to dance. As the people left, a small close friends and family went inside the house to continue drinking and chatting as dancing was impracticable in the small two room house that was built by Salema just after Touwa was born. Touwa's brothers and sisters were so kind to Dorisi; she was always seen smiling, as they explained as much as possible about the Salema family. Despite the good party, one by one left, and Dorisi and Touwa were getting an opportunity to rest after the long day of celebration.

On the day that followed, another invitation to eat drink and enjoy dancing at friend's home was repeated, and again on the next two days invitations kept on and on. On the fourth day, it was a period of rest and reflection on the love and respect that had been shown by family and friends alike. In the evening as Dorisi was kept busy talking with the cousins and nieces, Touwa was left alone. He sat on the 'kijiwe', the stone that was smooth, worn down by the many bottoms that sat there before him. Touwa thought about his life so far, especially the marriage and ceremony that was then coming to conclusion. He suddenly realised that he was then a man who had to take responsibilities. He thought of his large extended family, the wife who was then pregnant, the child, the care, the schooling and so the list kept on increasing. It was at that time that Touwa realised the enormity of his responsibilities that he exclaimed loudly and said *'the things that a man has to do'*, smiled and stood up to join Dorisi.

Salema, then aged 54, had promised a grand farewell to his son and his new daughter in law, with another party before they left for Dar es Salaam. That was the opportunity for Salema to give his son Touwa some adult advice and above all not to forget his folk. It was Salema classical party that included the drinking of *'mbege'*, meat eating, chatting and eventually singing that would end with the chorus of *'haya, o haya haya hee'* a chant that meant *'yes, oh yes, we fully agree'*.

Work at Keko Pharmaceutical plant:

Early in the morning, the newly weds took the early bus to Moshi town, then the long distant coach to Dar es Salaam.

At Dar es Salaam, the couple moved from Muhimbili to cousin Mtele's flat at Kariakoo. Touwa was also told that he was moving from Muhimbili to Keko Pharmaceutical plant where he was to be trained to lead the production team to complete the next six months of pre-registration. Touwa was happy both at home and for his new placement at Keko. That happy beginning helped Touwa to set up his goals more clearly, with a better outlook and building up his confidence for coping with family and work. Dorisi and Touwa settled well in their new flat with cousin Kipara and Moshiro who were studying at the local technical colleges. At Keko Pharmaceutical plant, Touwa was greeted by a Chinese's technical and pharmaceutical team who were the trainers and a young work force (average age was 22), who were the trainees. Touwa whose age was then 26 took i m m e n s e responsibility, forcing him to learn quick and to a high level with the ability to lead, solve p r o d u c t i o n

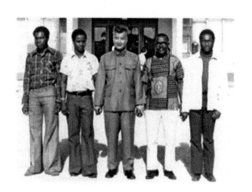

At Keko

problems, learn to order goods, time management in production schedules, solve dispute and even start modifications in order to improve some of the formulations. The smooth running of the Keko formulation plant that produced tablets and sterile intra venous solutions made Touwa a respectable leader of production to the young work force. The Chinese trainers were happy with Touwa's progress to an extent of increasing his responsibilities to manage the Pharmaceutical plant while reducing their roles to that of observers and advisers. The official opening of the Pharmaceutical plant by the then President of Tanzania J K Nyerere, marked the end of contract for the Chinese trainers, who left for China leaving Touwa as the production Manager, with a small team that included a Chemist to manage the quality control and an accountant to manage financial matters like salaries.

It was hard work for Touwa but there was a boost to his work when he discovered that some medicines he made at Keko were in use at the small dispensary in his home village

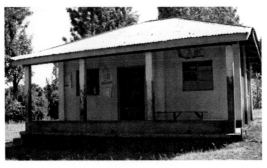

Local dispensary

Nanjara. That observation was used by Touwa as an example to all his staff when discussing product quality. He told his staff that failure to keep a high standard of quality was tantamount to a self inflicted death sentence. He clarified his statement by giving an example of a Keko worker who goes home to find his or her child sick, by taking the child to hospital, a poor quality medicine made in Keko to be administered resulting in a possible fatality! He asked who would be responsible for that outcome! The staff who

understood the question were silent, but replying by
nodding to show total agreement that they would be
responsible. With that accord of discipline and self regulating
mentality, Keko medicines were always of high quality when
tested by the bureau of standards of Tanzania and other
interested bodies. In addition to the respect he gained from
his staff, Touwa's reputation was also high at the Ministry of
Health, the owners and controllers of the pharmaceutical
plant. The Chief Pharmacist held Touwa with high esteem.
That respect enabled Touwa to give his opinion to the
Ministry of health on matters of hiring or firing, product
improvement or changes, tenders for orders and staff
benefits. Staff canteen with subsidizes lunch for staff was
one of the popular achievements that Touwa introduced to
Keko staff, giving him the opportunity to start a 24 hour
working day, that was accepted by all and worked efficiently.
Touwa's managerial skills were put to test when he succeeded
in providing enough vials of antibiotic injections and I V
fluids to be used in an outbreak of cholera. Touwa's humble
nature helped him to cope with the fame and great respect
he gained with senior officials at the Ministry of health.
Dorisi had learned a few word of the Swahili language; as a
result she was conversing with more people and was less
lonely when Touwa was away. A letter that Edith her mother
was not feeling well, prompted Dorisi to go to Birmingham.
With mutual agreement, she left for Birmingham to see her
mum, Edith, who was ill at that time. It was after Dorisi
had left that Touwa started to worry and feel lonely, as for a
whole year he had never been alone. Life however, was kept
cheerful with a stream of air mail letters between Dorisi and
Touwa. Touwa's life consisted of waiting for letters to read,
then replying and the work at Keko. The most exciting
letter was that reported the possible date of birth. That date

for the expected birth, came and passed and no letter was received. Touwa could not wait any longer, he wrote to ask what was happening. The waiting continued, Touwa's worries were noted by Kipara and Moshiro who lived with him in the flat. At work, Touwa confined his worries to his friend Fernandez, the accountant who reassured and calmed him. Moshiro and Kipara had to pass by the post office every day to check for incoming letters.

The baby:

One day in early December, a letter arrived; it was not the usual air mail letter but an envelope, rather firm to touch. With trembling hands, Touwa opened the letter to

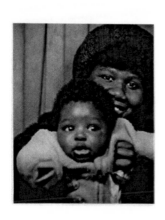

Mom and baby

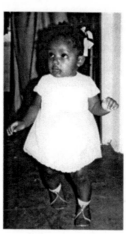

Heidi the baby

see two photographs, one a mother holding a baby and another of a baby, a girl! Kipara and Moshiro were also keen to see. *'She looks like you'*, they both cried in a chorus. It was the first time Touwa had realised the creation that was a product of his genes! He was ecstatic; he went to buy a hut and mittens for his daughter when she arrives in Dar es Salaam. That first born was immediately named Mkasu. That was the name of Touwa's mother, as tradition dictated; the first female born takes the name of the husband's mother. If the child was a boy, the name would have been Salema, the husbands father, while the second born would reflect in the wife's family as the Chagga tradition dictated. Touwa sat at the flats veranda, pondering the effect that new arrival to his family would bring. It was at that time he was reflecting that he fully realised he was a father, a husband, a family man and a working man. He could not think too much as Moshiro bought some beers and a mini celebration started.

The next day, Mkasu's picture was a source of congratulations from friends and staff of the Pharmaceutical plant. Dorisi and Touwa corresponded very frequently by airmail letter writing as access to international telephone call was neither cheap nor easy to obtain. The concept of mobile phones was then not known. Touwa's pass time became letter writing and waiting for Dorisi and Mkasu, to plan the travel to Dar es Salaam for Touwa to see, touch, and talk to his first born. The waiting was as if it was forever. A letter announcing the travelling plans for Mkasu and Dorisi became another reason to have a beer and a celebration. In Touwa's dreams were imaginations of what would happen the first time he sees his first born, a daughter. All that he imagined were the giggling, tickling, laughter and walking together to the shops, to friends and even to Keko. There were other important issues Touwa never thought about. He never imagined to make baby feed, to feed, to be woken up at night to feed or to clean and change nappy, to rush to the Doctor, to sing for her to stop crying and even to cool her when she was hot! Touwa realised all that he never thought about soon after the arrival of Mkasu.

On a sunny Sunday afternoon a roaring noise of Egypt air as it landed on the Dar es Salaam airport tarmac signified the arrival of Mkasu. Touwa and his friend Fernandez watched as the passengers came down the steps of the aircraft. A woman holding a baby appeared. She was wearing white blouse, white skirt and white shoes, holding a baby wrapped in a white shawl. Touwa lost his control as he shouted *'Dorisi, Dorisi, Dorisi'* until she heard him and waved! It was a short wait for checking passport and customs but to Touwa it appeared an eternity. Fernandez as usual reassured Touwa to calm down as the meeting was then to happen. As Touwa saw Dorisi through the glass doors, he called again. Dorisi moved closer to the Door and the guard allowed him to take the baby, to set Dorisi free to go to get the luggage.

With the baby, his daughter in his hands, you heard nothing but *'Mkasu, Mkasu, Mkasu, how are you'*. Touwa was talking so intensely to his baby daughter that he forgot about Fernandez and Dorisi. It was Fernandez who helped Dorisi with the luggage to the car to take the family to Kariakoo. Soon Touwa found what made the baby daughter laugh, and so the playing started. It was after a few giggling sessions that Touwa remembered Dorisi and asked how the journey was and had the chance of introducing Fernandez. Fernandez, a quiet gentleman, drove as if nothing was happening around him, as he gave Touwa the chance to get to know his first child, the daughter called Mkasu, and Dorisi, the wife who was curious observing father daughter bonding, with a hint of jealousy that she perceived and it appeared that she would be the second in line in Touwa's priorities. Fernandez indicated that they had arrived at the flat, as Moshiro and Kipara were waiting to welcome the new member of the household. Fernandez declined to join the family, as he left due to other commitments. Moshiro had prepared a small party to welcome Dorisi and Mkasu who were very tired and it did not take long before they went to sleep. Dorisi, however did not sleep until she told Touwa a bit about the birth of his daughter. After a long labour pain at 00.02 hours on the 29th October 1975, the child was born. After more stories she fell asleep. It was the next day that Touwa tried on the hat and mittens he bought when she was born, to find they were too small attracting laughter from Dorisi indicating that Touwa had no idea about dressing a baby. That was the start of Touwa's learning curve on matters concerning babies and family. The baby, Mkasu was developing well, starting to crawl, attempts to stand and as days passed she was on two feet, running and causing chaos in the flat. The active child prompted Touwa to think of a better place that would enable the child to play more freely. In order to relocate he applied for a house but he got a ground floor flat, that had ample area to play. The flat at Upanga near Muhimbili hospital, was a residential place with less traffic noise and dust. That was Touwa's own first family home. It was at that flat the family grew up, become a place where there was happiness and sometimes sad occasions, crying moments, some moody times but above all there was plenty of laughter.

An addition to the family:

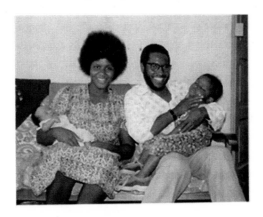

Touwa family

It was during residing at that flat Touwa's younger brother Melikoi joined the family from Arusha. Melikoi joined cousin Kipara who was studying vocational training in refrigeration and repair of fridges. Melikoi studied tool making. When they finished they found jobs and became independent of Touwa. It was also in that flat that a second child, a boy was born, instantly nicknamed Hagaly by her sister, Mkasu, although his name would have been Salema, to mirror his grandfather, the name Hagaly was accepted and used. Mkasu used the name *'haangalii'* a Swahili word which meant *'he is not looking'* as the child' eyes

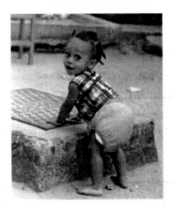

Hagaly baby

were closed when the little girl saw him first, but her mother who spoke less of Swahili than Mkasu thought she said Hagaly. Hagaly born at 14.28 hours on 27th August 1977, a Saturday afternoon, he was cute and handsome. His high level of intelligence and an acute sense of surroundings observed during the infancy were proved correct when he was able to stand and walk at the age of nine months with the ability to mimic whatever he heard from radio, or mimic chats of people talking in the streets. At age one he talked fluently and intelligently speaking the local Swahili language. With then two children, Touwa was a happy married man with respect at his work.

That level of contentment was the trigger for Touwa to try to find a hobby, notably gardening. The first garden was done on a patch in front of their ground floor flat, on which a fast growing green vegetables known locally as *'mchicha'* was grown. It was the good taste of the fresh vegetable that prompted Touwa to think bigger!

The visit to Mbezi:

That big thought had the chance to be put into reality when a good neighbour gave Touwa some fresh bananas! In acceptance Touwa asked where she obtained such sweet and fresh bananas. The reply to Touwa's quest led to the introduction of an area 20 Km outside Dar es Salaam called Mbezi. One Sunday morning,

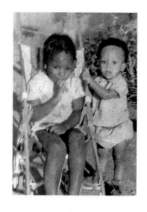

Mkasu and hagaly in Dar

160

Touwa travelled to Mbezi to see the possibility of getting a small plot to plant some food crops. In the process of finding the land Touwa learned that there was plenty of land and there was an encouragement to build and settle if one desired. With two childrenand the responsibilities, it was not hard to convince Touwa to desire a piece of land to grow fresh food. When Touwa got a 2.5 hector piece of land that he started to plant all sorts of food plants ranging from corn, beans, rice, bananas, including *'mchicha'* (green leafy

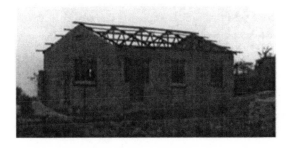

Mbezi house in construction

vegetable)to tomatoes. A wish to build a house on the land that he had acquired was boosted by the government announcement of establishing a mortgage system where money to build a house could be borrowed and repaid over a number of years. Touwa promptly took that opportunity, got a mortgage and aspired to build his own first house. The plans were made, the logistics of obtaining building materials were in place, but Touwa was in fear of failure, so he took some time before collecting the first mortgage instalment. It was during that thinking time that Touwa's brother Melikoi, returned from Mwanza to Dar es Salaam to look for better opportunities, when Touwa confided in him the house building plans. Melikoi was so excited, encouraged a speedy start, and offered to help.

The Mbezi house 1978:

Architectural plans for a three bedroom bungalow, with kitchen, lounge with shower and toilet facilities was made. Prior to starting the construction Salema's approval was requested and was granted. It was then that a local builder was hired to start construction. The building progress was very slow because work was done at weekends only due to many commitments of the key workers. The slow work raised some problems like bulk buying, storage and theft of some construction materials. In addressing these problems, a wooden hut was made and a guard was employed, that was when Mashaka met Touwa. Mashaka

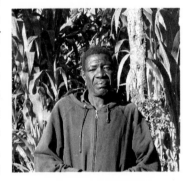

Mashaka adopted son

became trusted, and eventually became friends with Touwa, Ndesumbuka and Melikoi, then later became a helper to Salema and eventually he was adopted as a family member. As a family member he was given a land to build a house and raise his family among the many of Salema's children at Nanjara. It was during the construction of the Mbezi house in 1978 that many things that influenced the family of Salema occurred.

It was when Melikoi, who was working at a bicycle manufacturing plant while at weekends helping Touwa to build the house, made a glimpse of a girl who later became his wife. Ndesumbuka, Touwa's brother, casually came to Dar es Salaam, not sure where his brother Touwa lived, but as he checked the street he saw a cousin Kipara who knew where Touwa's house was. Ndesumbuka had then finished his high school studies, in 1975, worked as a bus conductor, then as a teacher but was aspiring to go to university. The meeting of the two brothers was significant because Ndesumbuka started teaching work in Dar es Salaam schools, then he got a technician job at Keko pharmaceutical plant, joined a college Of business Education studying Legal Metrology, and eventually got a scholarship the following year to study Geology in the then USSR, although he acquired a degree of masters in Pharmacy. His original aim of visiting his brother in Dar es Salaam was only to borrow some money to buy a gear box for his van as at that time he was aspiring to be a business man on transportation.

When Shenji was 108 years old:

It was also the year that Shenji the beloved grandfather to Touwa, Ndesumbuka and Melikoi including many more, passed away aged 108 years. He was an inspiration to Touwa as well as to his many grandchildren. He championed education, self respect and independence. He had a keen understanding of the pains of growing up, by showing sympathy and offering words of encouragement and comfort. He celebrated by slaughtering a sheep or goat for the smallest happy incident that his grandchildren encountered like passing exams, welcoming home from boarding school or when he observed hard work in the family's *'shamba'*. Shenji, the beloved grandfather, took special attention to having quality time with his grandchildren, especially those who were in schools, when they visited during their holidays. At one time during such holidays, he saw Ndesumbuka with a girl. He was glad to see that his grandchildren were mixing properly with their friends. One day when Shenji was eating with his grandchildren, the usual practice he performed after a sheep slaughter, he uttered his famous words:

'mndu mfele kakuninga, ambwa utale e namu tewete chafo'

In these famous granddad's words he was telling his grandchildren who were then becoming young men to respect and treat women good as that was the root towards success in life. Broadly speaking he meant that one should not be conceited as to refuse to love someone who shows an interest in love as happiness cannot be achieved by keeping alone. Before Shenji died, he advised that attending to a funeral for family was a very good act but for those who were far away at work or studies, it should not be a must. That order helped to reduce blaming those who fail to attend family funerals. Those words showed that Shenji had a vision that many of his grandchildren would probably live far from one another or even in different countries. That was because he perceived the problems of urgency in travel, work constrains or finances that may not coincide with funeral arrangements. That was a hint to the grandchildren who were far away that they should come to pay their respects when he died but without causing undue disruption to their work or family life. Shenji's ideas and efforts that helped to keep his family united were continued by his son Salema.

It was also that year that two promises were made. Melikoi promised Touwa that he would move into the house as soon as the roof was set. Salema then 58 years old, appeared an old man by his children promised that he would travel to go to Dar es Salaam to see the house. Kimwai, Touwa's uncle secured that promise from Salema who had not travelled away from Kilimanjaro region since he got married, 37 years ago. The pressure that Salema would visit the Mbezi house made Melikoi work hard to plant bananas that bore large bunches as big a Touwa's daughter Mkasu He made 'mbege' ready for his father's visit.

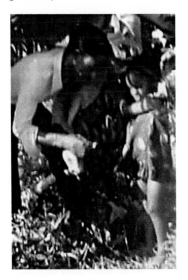

Mkasu at Mbezi farm

That same year, demand for medicines formulated at Keko was high such that the Health Ministry asked Touwa to look at possibilities of production increase and diversification. In order to write a complete report, Touwa utilised the services of lecturers at the department of

Pharmacy, the newly qualified Pharmacists from Muhimbili, and all the staff at Keko for ideas prior to writing his plans on plant expansion and diversification. The quality and depth of the plans caught the eye of the then Health Minister Dr Sterling, who called Touwa for a face to face meeting to elucidate further on the practicability of the plans. The ability to explain and answer the many questions convinced the Minister and the Directors to accept and promise to present it to government department for analysis and financial projections.

Touwa was not privileged to see the new equipment, or how productivity was affected, as he got a W.H.O. (World Health Organisation)scholarship that year to study at Aston University in Birmingham. Professor Wibberley had recommended Touwa for research studies in Pharmaceutics. With a good record of work at Keko, the Ministry of Health granted the scholarship to Touwa. In November 1978, Touwa left Tanzania for studies in UK for the second time. It was the year that Uganda invaded Tanzania in an act of war. That war brought about a detrimental effect to the economy of Tanzania with effects that could not have been predicted or even comprehended.

CHAPTER 8

Leaving Keko for advanced studies

Touwa's preparation to leave for studies was very difficult as the country was at war. First duty was to find a suitable successor to lead the production of medicines at Keko Pharmaceutical plant. Second he had to make speedy travel arrangements, like vaccinations and his sons travel documents to ensure arrival at the University at the planned time. The war also made it difficult to get quick internal travel plans. The combination of such events led to Touwa leaving Tanzania without having the chance to see his father or daughter Mkasu at Nanjara. Touwa travelled with Hagali. The building of the Mbezi house was left to the brothers Ndesumbuka and Melikoi to finish. All the travelling plans were done in a hurry as the reporting at Aston University was by a set date for the scholarship to be honoured. Flying with air France, to Paris with connection to London was as smooth as it could be as the baby Hagali, who was at that time 13 months old did not suffer any flight problems, like flight sickness, panic or crying. At the transit launch in the airport at Paris, Hagali was happy running around fast in the huge space. Touwa had difficulty running to catch him. His charm made many people talk and showed the need to hold and be with him but he was too active to stay in one place without something to do. At Heathrow airport, a compatriot who heard Touwa and Hagali conversing in Swahili, offered to give a lift to the train station where he also bought Hagali a toy dog.

Touwa a student again:

In Birmingham Touwa was in familiar surroundings and it was no trouble taking a taxi to see Dorisi who had left earlier to attend to her mother who was then sick. Arrangements to find housing started immediately and two days later Dorisi, Touwa and Hagali were moving to a very cold flat at St Peter's road in Handsworth. Work at Aston University started immediately under the supervision of the then Dr Irwin and Dr Li wan Po who carried the wishes of Pro Wibberley who was the source and inspiration of the WHO scholarship. The family was re united as Mkasu

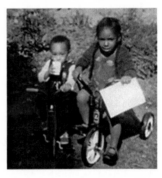

Mkasu and hagaly in brum

was collected by Dorisi, and all were happy. Life was the usual combination of work, study, and family activities coupled with a move to a new warmer flat at Highfield road in Moseley where Dorisi and the children lived during the whole of the study period.

It was during the years at Highfield road that Touwa passed his driving test, bought his first car, then bought bicycles for his children, and start taking his children to school. As the father and children were going to school each morning, Dorisi commented that it was comic that dad and children were going to school together.

Ndesumbuka's travels:

It was also during that period (1979-1985)at that address, that Ndesumbuka who was then studying in USSR visited Touwa's family. The one memorable event in that first visit, which was one of many, he travelled from Zaporozhye to UK by train and ferryboat. In Germany he bought a cooked chicken, well wrapped as a gift to his brother and family. From Berlin to Birmingham he used the train, a ferryboat then the train again. At Birmingham train station he took a taxi by showing the taxi driver the address

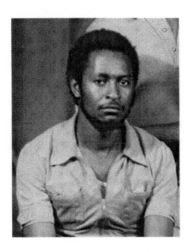

Ndesumbuka days in ussr

that was flat 3 number sixteen Highfield road. Flat three was upstairs, accessed through an external door which was downstairs. A neighbour at flat two let in Ndesumbuka into the door of flat three. He knocked the door for hours with no reply. He decided to sleep in front of the door marked flat no 3. That night Dorisi was working. Touwa, Mkasu and Hagali were asleep, and no one heard the knock until morning when preparations to go to school were made for Mkasu. In the morning just before Dorisi arrived, a knock

169

at the door prompted Mkasu to call her dad to open the door when a mighty loud *'good morning brother'* was heard. As Ndesumbuka entered the warmer surroundings, he was having a warm cup of coffee when Dorisi arrived. After greetings, Ndesumbuka opened his bag to give each person their presents he had bought. The last was a present for the family. That was a roast chicken, which Ndesumbuka thought could supplement breakfast. He opened the first wrapping, a little whiff of smell was detected but on opening the second wrapping, the stench was overpowering such that Dorisi threw it in the dust-bin but the dust-bin continued stinking so much that the whole flat stunk. The whole dust-bin with contents was thrown outside, all windows were open and that became a topic of conversation for several years as the children referred to it as "*uncle's stinky chicken*". That first journey of Ndesumbuka to UK was one of many he made until he left USSR after his studies. It was also during that period a reciprocal visit was done to USSR by Touwa and Dorisi.

At Moscow airport, a large land mass almost hidden from view by an elaborate forest of tall trees that surrounded it, Touwa and his wife were received by Ndesumbuka who could read and speak Russian language fluently. A travel visa form one town to another was required to enable the taking of the overnight train journey to Zaporozhye where Ndesumbuka was studying. The town lies along the banks of the mighty Dnieper River that flows to the Sea of Azov, a very popular health-resort area that eventually joins to the Black sea 150-200 km away. Life in Zaporozhye was spent at student residences, accompanied by many of Ndesumbuka's female and male friends, who were very hospitable and friendly to a level that they invited Touwa and Dorisi to their parents' homes. After two weeks of socializing, drinking vodka and sight seeing, it was time to return to Moscow and fly to London. The train journey was during the day, an opportunity to see the Russian country that consisted of large farms, very few residential areas and lots of forests At Moscow Touwa, Ndesumbuka and Dorisi checked into a hotel for the night, in preparation for the flight the following day. Sight seeing in Moscow led Ndesumbuka and his guests to a shopping mall. It was large, with many goods, some Russian made but the western made goods were very expensive. Walking in Moscow was not a very pleasant experience as Dorisi expressed that she felt constantly being watched. At the mall a need to go to the toilet, made the visitors find out that the toilets were not fitted with doors! Touwa had to stand on the door to protect Dorisi while using the loo! It was not clear if that was part of watching and security. In the afternoon prior to leaving Moscow, Ndesumbuka took his brother to a buffet with good food, but the best of that food was that described as fish soup that Dorisi found it so tasty and exquisite. That holiday marked the conclusion of Touwa's studies for an award of a Doctor of Philosophy degree in Pharmaceutical Sciences, for the award of the higher Doctorate degree.

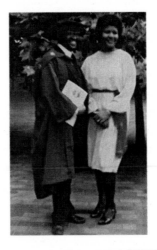

Touwa with dorisi at graduation

An addition to the family:

To qualify as a practising Pharmacist in UK, Touwa underwent a 12 months pre registration training that he completed and started working as a community Pharmacist. It was during the training period that the family was blessed with the birth of the third child, a boy. At Sorrento Maternity hospital, in a cold winter night at 21.16 hours on the 13th February 1983, the boy, Siti, was born. (*Pictured in the middle of Sister Mkasu and bother Hagali*)His joints used to make some clicking noises, the parents called him 'Rackety' but that nick name did not last as the condition was over swiftly. On his regular annual summer visits to UK, Ndesumbuka took the duties of baby sitting Siti. It was during Ndesumbuka's

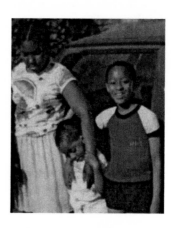

The kids3

travels from Moscow to Birmingham and the baby sitting sessions at the family home of his brother Touwa that the two brothers chatted about life at home, that Ndesumbuka had a lot to tell, starting with his education in high school and in Russia or the then USSR.

Ndesumbuka's diary:

It was during such meetings of the brothers that they got a unique opportunity to relate to one another their life events as recalled by Ndesumbuka. The events started from the moment the two brothers met in Dar es Salaam some years back. There was lots of talk as the two brothers had been apart in most of their schooldays. Ndesumbuka finished high school in 1975 at Muhoho, in Kenya. Due to various problems in the study years Ndesumbuka and a very close friend Gathena, were in tears when they left Muhoho thinking they had failed. Ndesumbuka had problems with school authorities such that he was nearly expelled while Gathena's dad had died a few months back. Despite their thoughts that they would fail, the two friends promised each other that they would struggle even to get '*the simplest degree on earth*' a promise that would always prompt them to aspire for higher things in life. The two months that followed, the results were out and the two friends passed well but Gathena got a place in Nairobi University for a degree of BSc in education. The two friends' pathways became very different as Ndesumbuka did not get a university place. That was the start of Ndesumbuka trying various jobs like working as a conductor in buses, then as a teacher in a girls school and finally as an owner of a mini bus, the gear box, problems led him to travel to Dar es Salaam to meet his older brother Touwa. The possibility of more opportunities in the capital city Dar es Salaam encouraged Ndesumbuka to stay. Touwa helped by securing a temporary job at Keko Pharmaceutical plant. Ndesumbuka increased his income by securing a second job teaching. It was when Ndesumbuka was working that hard, in addition to building the Mbezi house that Touwa got his scholarship and left for his higher studies abroad. The following year, Gathena, Ndesumbuka's high school friend graduated with a BSc in Education. When Ndesumbuka heard of his friend's fulfilling the promise they had made, he was consumed with constructive jealousy, anger and determination to go for that simple degree! He started looking in newspapers, by applying to various offices and contacting known friends for educational opportunities. When he was at field work as a student in Legal Metrology, he heard in the radio broadcast the names of students selected to study in the 'USSR'. Urgent reporting to the Ministry of education, getting passport, stipend and Aeroflot tickets within two weeks was not a small task. But Ndesumbuka was so determined to succeed as his friend Gathena had done. When Ndesumbuka found himself with friends on a flight from Dar es Salaam to Moscow he was thrilled, that he had achieved his goal, *'to get even the smallest degree!* At Moscow students were dispersed to various institutes for language studies that were geared for the aspired degree. Ndesumbuka and a new friend Mutiba were posted to Zaporozhye Medical Institute in preparation for degrees of Pharmacy and Medicine. Ndesumbuka, however, was aspiring to study Geology; unfortunately the authorities were not aware of that until at the end of the language year. After that year, Ndesumbuka's group had to proceed to do either Medicine or Pharmacy. As it was mandatory to do another language year in order to do Geology, Ndesumbuka wisely opted for Pharmacy and it was as a Pharmacist he graduated in 1985 with a degree of MSc in Pharmacy, *'not the smallest degree'* as the two friends had vowed to achieve. With that note of success Ndesumbuka did not forget the suffering he endured with his bothers Tabu, Tabuni and Melikoi in the hands of Mamoroi and seeing his father unable to do anything.

Ndesumbuka, Melikoi, Tabu and Tabuni plights:

Tabu and Tabuni were very young when their mother Mkasu passed away. It was when they found themselves under the authority of a step mother and that they were then old enough to know that all in the family was not well. The first things the boys observed that was there was bias in the treatment of the children under her care they received, that was; Mamoroi's children got the best care while Mkasu's children had total lack of care. That was strikingly evident when Mamoroi gave birth to a fourth child. The older child Ndesumbuka started to rebel to protect his brothers. He became the nucleus that the hatred was focused. That hatred resulted in a block punishment to Mkasu's children that went on for several years. They were segregated, they fended for themselves. Ndesumbuka, Tabu and Tabuni had to cook their own food, find the food first, fetch water, chop wood, cleaning their school uniforms, buy kerosene for their lantern that provided some light in their hut, and above all go to school. It was like a camp, the three boys had to unite, as Melikoi had left to live with his teacher. They coined their dwellings, KMA (*Kambi ya Manyani*)translated to 'Camp of Monkeys'. It was a kind of association that helped to bond, unite and strengthen the boys in their struggle to survive and a determination to attain education that they believed would be a saviour because it was not easy to survive in such hatred, isolation, neglect and total lack of care when so young. Despite the odds, the association designed survival plans that helped the boys in their struggle of getting food and other essentials. Salema was under intense pressure but he encouraged the three suffering boys to go to school, as in his wisdom he thought, if they passed the camp would be a temporary issue, as they would go away as Touwa did. That was the time Touwa was in the University and he sent few presents to his family that probably gave Salema hope that there could be a better future. Hope was realised when Ndesumbuka passed and went to Olkejuado Secondary school leaving his two brothers in the camp. Two years later Tabu followed him to

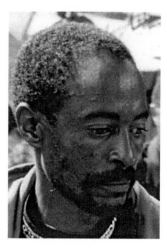

Tabuni

the same school. Tabuni however, did not pass to go to secondary school he returned to live with Yohana the grandmother where he found acceptance and started to learn how to do business. Salema had a great burden of school fees payment on his shoulders. He had to pay fees for the two boys and could not do any more. Melikoi who was staying with his teacher to avoid the KMA dwellings, was forced go to Arusha to find employment after completion of his primary education. Mamoroi's children did not pass to go to secondary school some did not like school at all, so they stayed with their mother. Touwa was working for a brief moment a period when he bought presents to Salema and Mamoroi and the children without exception. That act was probably the gesture that led to a change of attitudes as Salema started to be assisted with his wife in the education of the two boys.

The change of attitude was confirmed by Tabu when he arrived home to find the camp abandoned because no one was in it. When he asked for the pots to cook his food he was asked to wait and instead of pots, Tabu was given food by Mamoroi. That act of being given food and accepting it was a start of near normal family relationship. Mamoroi had proved her respect to Tabu. Mamoroi was ill for a while. It was when she was ill that Tabu graduated. Although she was very ill she insisted on going to the graduation of Tabu.

She was showing concern to Tabu's future and was eager to see his marriage to Kavengi. Mamoroi died in 1986 leaving eight children, five girls and three boys. Tabu and Kavengi both with diplomas in Education got married in 1991 and had five children

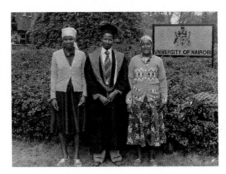

Garaduation of Tabu

Sani, Mato (a girl), Ketukei, Lenkoya and Lemaiyan. Tabu aimed higher and studied to attain a degree in Education—BA in Education with children that fast followed the footsteps of their mum and dad.

Mamoroi, the step mother:

The escape to the boundary farm eased Salema's women problems. His hard working ethics helped him in gaining the confidence and some respect from his wives and he was becoming happy again. When tragedy hit, Salema's life was again in turmoil. The sudden death of his first wife, forced him to be a single parent looking after his children alone without Mkasu. For reasons not clear to anyone Salema hated Nanjara, the home he had left for the boundary farm, and started to make new friend. It was during social

occasions with the new neighbours that Mamoroi caught
Salema's eye or may be the vice versa. In less than two years
Mamoroi started to visit Salema at his hut and going home,
then an overnight stay and eventually a resident. The duty
of care for Mkasu's boys was reluctantly accepted and that
reluctance was evident when she had her own children.
Mamoroi was a tall slim woman about five feet, three
inches (1.58 metres)with a pleasant radiant smile which was
evident for those she liked. When she was angry there was
a clear indication of her mood. The total lack of care that
followed for Mkasu's boys was described in Tabu's plight, as
it affected Ndesumbuka, Melikoi, Tabu and Tabuni. The
KMA (Kambi *ya Manyani*)was their bond that enabled
them to achieve survival that lasted until the boys were
grown ups. The grown up Mkasu's children left home to
various schools. When they returned home for holidays,
they never showed animosity to Mamoroi and above all were
able to bring her presents. There was a significant change in
the behaviour of Mamoroi towards Mkasu's children. For
reasons that cannot easily be pin-pointed, Mamoroi showed
care and even love that was in evidence through her actions.
She insisted in going to Tabu's graduation and even bought
a cow in partnership with Touwa to enhance her wealth.
When she was ill, it was Ndesumbuka who took her to Dar
es Salaam to get treatment in the main hospital. When she
died in 1986 aged 44 years she had gained the love of all.

CHAPTER 9

As the Years Passed

The growing family:

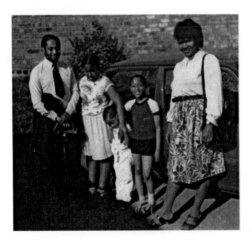

Touwas family

The life of Touwa was improving after graduating, getting registered as a Pharmacist in UK and securing work with Bannister and Thatcher Chemists Ltd. Dorisi was also working in the NHS hospital, their income enabled them to take a mortgage for a three bedroom town house. It was in that house that Ndesumbuka stayed during his visits from USSR. Mkasu and Hagali were then in school, their father and mother were working constantly to afford the mortgage and improve their standards of life while looking after the baby, Siti. It was for about six weeks every summer holiday for four years that Ndesumbuka became a baby sitter to Siti, making him the '*most welcome visitor*'. Dorisi worked nights, and baby-sit in the day while Touwa worked during the day to baby-sit at nights, an arrangement that worked perfect until the need was not necessary with passing time. Touwa worked even harder as he acquired his Pharmacy named: Mroso Dispensing Chemist. Self employed, as it was at that time was a tough life for Touwa who worked without a break for four years. A good friend Mrs Patterson and confidant stirred Touwa during the tough periods by helping, mentoring and encouragement. That was a friend indeed.

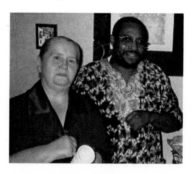

Nell and Touwa

Touwa and Dorisi endured the trials of life like most people, but they had particular joy in their work, their children who were healthy and growing up well, their house, good friends and financially secure, as they could pay their mortgage and take short breaks. It was not always that sweet but tears were shed sometimes like when theft threatened their business or when the children as teens expressed their opinions too forcefully, causing worry. Issues like non—attendance to school or not returning from school caused lots of stress. Dorisi and Touwa had their fair share of worry for their children; it was like hell on earth. Life was very slow, day by day not knowing what the next day brought. The saying that *'time heals'* may have applied in that period because as the children grew older, they re-discovered respect. When they left home, they met *'responsibility'* a thing that gave them the shock in their early life. That shock forced them to reflect on those home comforts missed and so *'respect to mum and dad was re-discovered'.* The return of mutual discussions and advice were the first steps that the children were making progress *'glee, tears and years'* in their lives was shouldered by themselves instead of their parents.

Mkasu developed into a beautiful young woman with great future expectations. She worked in a shoe shop *'Clarks'* where she bought her father exceedingly good fitting shoes. It was unfortunate she did not continue in that line of work but after her family was more independent she aspired to study in order to teach young children.

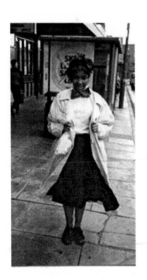

Mkasu at 18

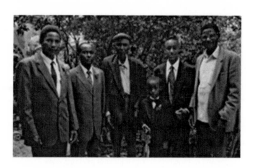

Hagaly with Salema, and uncles

Hagali aged thirteen was pictured with his grandad, Salema, when he made a visit to Africa for uncle Melikoi's wedding. He studied to become an IT engineer in network solutions. That career path was noted at the early stage in primary school when he was able to set up the school sound system and proved handy with tool when he made a model Viking ship that survived the weather elements outside the garden until it was photographed 27 years later when Hagaly was over 33 years old.

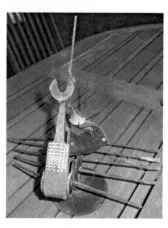

Anthony's vicking ship

Siti the youngest, aimed to study to become a graduate and followed a career of teaching sports science and mathematics. That level of discipline started when he used to monitor his father's driving to ensure that he did not go over the speed limit. If that happened he reported to his mother promptly. With similar discipline, he landed his father Touwa on the headmaster's office charged with driving through a red light as reported by Siti. The Headmaster, Mr Matthews, a family friend, reprimanded Touwa in front of his son emphasizing on showing good example. As a grown up, a teacher as a career, Siti has to be an example to many.

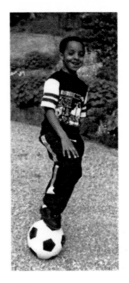

Siti as sportsman

Touwa's Children:

Mkasu, the first child, was born in Birmingham *(Queen Elizabeth Hospital)*at the time when Touwa was in Dar es Salaam. It was six months later that Touwa saw her.

Hagali was born in Dar es Salaam *(Aga Khan Hospital)*. Touwa was away in Belgium. Just before his birth Touwa went for a study tour to Belgium hoping he would be back for the birth. It was at the airport that his friend Fernando, shouted, *"it is a boy"* as Touwa was descending down the steps of the Belgian airline, Sabena. He was glad that he then had a girl and a boy in his family. It was a fast drive from the airport to his residence at Upanga to hold his two day old son.

It was a privilege that Touwa was present to witness his son Siti's birth. Touwa had to travel from London to Birmingham on a cold winter evening when Dorisi told him to be home for the birth. Touwa vowed never to miss that birth like he had done for the other two kids. At the hospital in Moseley *(Sorrento Maternity),* late in the night the boy was born. When Dorisi was in stress, Touwa asked the midwife if he could go outside, as he did not like to see the suffering, the groaning and the breathing. The midwife held Touwa's arm saying,

"You are not going anywhere you will see it through so sit."

When the baby was born, and all was well, the midwife told Doris that Touwa was about to faint. Dorisi told Siti when he was grown up that his dad fainted when he was born, a joke that dad had to endure.

The marriage of Sesilia to Oyeko:

Sitting down in their sitting room in front of the fireplace, while the kids, Mkasu, Hagali and Siti were upstairs, Dorisi answered to the ringing of the door bell. On opening the door it was her niece Sesilia, hand in hand with a young man, Oyeko. It was not a shock to Dorisi as she had seen the pair together a few days earlier but that day at the house it was for a formal introduction. It was after a cup of tea and biscuits that Sesilia asked the auntie if she could help in organizing a wedding, as the couple had decided to get married. That was not a shock as Sesilia was in her 30's. Dorisi's brain started racing with plans and ideas, like clothes food, photographs, reception

184

hall and many things that organising a wedding requires. The list was becoming huge so Dorisi in an attempt to reduce her list she asked some questions to assess the level of preparedness and the depth of planning. *'When do you plan the wedding day?'* Dorisi asked. *'Three weeks'* was the definite answer from Sesilia. Dorisi was in shock as she knew that weddings were planned over periods counted by years and months not weeks and days. The shock prompted her to ask more questions like, invitations, plans of food and drinks, venue, catering, bridesmaids, cakes, flowers and even if any other members of the family knew. When all the answers were either *'no or don't know'*, Dorisi's frustration was apparent and she remarked: *Aren't you cutting it fine?'* Although Touwa who was sitting next to Dorisi did not fully grasp the meaning of the remark, tried to promote progress in the talks by suggesting to the couple to put everything pertaining to the wedding as a list on a piece of paper, with a view to meet the following day to allocate tasks and prepare a timetable. As soon as the couple left, Dorisi and Touwa entered into a stage of hyper-activity of contacts and information seeking. Anastasia, was first to be contacted as she makes exceedingly good cakes but above all she excels in catering for small and large groups. The two sisters, Dorisi and Anastasia made all the catering plans over the phone, even before the couple's plans were known. The high speed that plans had to be implemented meant that planning stage was cut to the minimum, to allow practical tasks and activities to commence. That need prompted Anastasia to drive to Birmingham with her husband Jonii, a distance of 193.6 Km to meet Dorisi, Sesilia, Oyeko and Touwa to finalise the wedding plans. It was a mutual agreement to hold another meeting in three days time to see how each team had put plans to practice and the financial standing to cover the costs. The meeting time at Touwa's house did not go smoothly due to delays by the couple. At the meeting it was realised that the couple had not made any plans and above all appear to know very little in planning a wedding ceremony. They had however printed nice invitation cards for a large number of people but had no clue to the amount of food or drinks needed or even the size of the reception hall. The poor level of understanding that the couple portrayed made Dorisi rather annoyed but determined to make it a success as it was a wedding for her favourite niece. Dorisi took charge and told the couple the essential tasks they had to complete before sending them away with her non complementing remark: *'you really have cut it fine so get moving'* When they both answered *'thank you'* Dorisi knew that they did not understand the irony of the remark! When the couple left, Dorisi, Anastasia, Jonii and Touwa got into serious brain storming on all matters pertaining to planning for a wedding, from food or transport to the wedding day schedule of events. As the days moved closer to the wedding day check were constantly being made by Dorisi and Touwa to ensure desirable progress was achieved. Food preparation started three days before the wedding day because the food had to be as fresh as possible, second storage in a family set up was limited and thirdly there were only two main cooks, Anastasia, the chef, Dorisi the assistant while the men Touwa and Jonii, the husbands, became the errand boys, to fetch and deliver all that the chef wanted. The children were not spared the hard work. They constantly helped in cleaning, sweeping or polishing in accordance to what the chefs deemed as needed. Mkasu who was then sixteen helped more while Hagali and Siti found it all amusing seeing adults so busy and tense. The level of pressure was manifested by an urgent need of a large cooking pot that was 193.6 Km away at Anastasia's house. Touwa and Jonii had to drive to collect that pot at an expense that exceeded the cost of the pot. The day before the wedding, cooking started in earnest. More hands were needed for helping in chores like cutting onions or making salads. Touwa sought help from friends who were currently students at the University. East African students who were pleased to help were Asha and Sewe from Kenya, Sara from Tanzania, Halima from Zanzibar and Mangeni from Uganda. The five girls worked hard as they succeeded in preparing the seasoning and vegetables that were used in various dished for the wedding. Early morning of Saturday, the wedding day, it had been arranged that the hair dresser would come to style the hair for the women, but the hair dresser was so late that the African girls who had come early to continue with their help turned to help in hair dressing. The plan was for the bride to come, to dress, and to proceed to the registry, chauffeured by Touwa. The wedding time at the registry was eleven o'clock. At ten o'clock, the bride was just starting to get ready and the hair was not done. Everyone was working frantically to make to the registry at eleven. Anastasia and the African girls decided not to go to the registry in order to ensure that food would be on time and to free the bathroom use for the few who were going to the registry. The car was not well decorated so the girls also helped to put a ribbon and some flowers. It was quarter to eleven; Touwa was worried whether he would reach the registry in time. In a loud voice he called his wife Dorisi to grab the bride, ready or not to go or else they would be late, as late arrival means losing one's marriage oath slot with a possibility of delay or postponement. Almost immediately the bride entered into the car and Touwa sped to the registry. Due to the delay Touwa who had a minute grace when he arrived at the registry could not waste more time looking for a parking spot so he stopped next to a pedestrian crossing. That was a serious mistake because as he stopped for the bride to get out, a Police officer approached the car and ordered the driver to move immediately. At that very moment the bride was getting out of the car slowly checking if hair, dress or flowers were ok. The Police officer was getting irate as Touwa could not move the car as the bride had one foot on the tarmac. *'Move it'* the policeman said again in a very stern voice. Touwa in turn shouted to Dorisi, *'what are you doing, I must move'.* Without patience Policeman started to write a ticket but at that moment the back door was shut allowing Touwa to drive fast from the spot leaving the irate policeman and narrowly avoiding a booking. After the marriage oath, the bride and groom were driven to their house to take pictures before proceeding to the hall where the reception was to be held.

Jonii and Touwa went to the hall to check whether the promised setup was done, to find that the hall was neither opened nor decorated. One option was to start cleaning, dusting, arranging tables and decorating. The catering people brought the cutlery, but the music set up, decorators and flowers were not seen until an hour before reception time and that was after a series of heated telephone calls. Drinks and food was collected and with luck all was well by four o'clock when the bride was to make an entry into the hall. Guests were given a drink as they arrived, were shown a place to sit and they enjoyed the music. After four Anastasia arrived at the hall to organize the catering. All the food and drinks had been collected from Touwa's house to the hall. When the bride and groom arrived, the hall atmosphere came to life, music, chatting, singing, greetings, congratulations and a number of witty speeches that made all the guests relax and enjoy a drink. The late entry of the

African relatives of the groom, with drums, waist wiggling and bum shaking dancing and singing made the reception a memorable occasion radiating happiness to all the guests. The celebrations went on past midnight when tiredness forced one by one of the guest to say their goodbyes and retire to their warm beds. When Anastasia and Dorisi arrived home, concluded it was a success, Jonii agreed but Touwa remembered the joke, *'didn't they cut it fine?'* Dorisi was glad to see Touwa who hardly understood sarcasms was trying to utter one.

Salema's Birmingham visit:

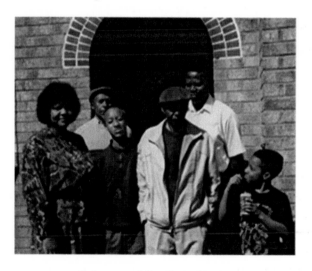

Salema and family in brum

A year after Sesilia and Oyeko's wedding Touwa took a bold step to invite his father to Birmingham, envisaging no unforeseen problems. Salema, Touwa's father, was then 71 years old when his son asked if he could travel to Birmingham to see his grandchildren. The idea of travelling leaving his house, in fear of the forest swallowing or engulfing it by overgrowth, taking a plane, the small flying object in the sky, and the idea of leaving Nanjara after such a long period of non-travel, made Salema to categorically say *'no'* to the invitation. The determination that his father should travel drove Touwa to use the persuasive abilities of brother Ndesumbuka, cousin Lazaro and uncle Kimwai. The friendship of Kimwai and Salema with son Ndesumbuka and the help from the great friend and cousin Lazaro set to work to change Salema's mind. In addition it was planned that Kimwai and Lazaro would accompany him, the sweetest incentive for hard work. When they succeeded they made it possible for Salema to travel on board a British airways direct flight from Nairobi to arrive London on a sunny Sunday afternoon in July. It was the first time Salema and Touwa had met outside Kilimanjaro. The emotional re union at the airport blocked the arrivals exit for a moment as Touwa, Salema, Siti, Kimwai, Lazaro and Runyoro hugged one another with exceptional happiness. It was the first time Salema experienced driving on motorway speeds and above all by his own son on the way from London to Birmingham. The picture above shows Dorisi, Kimwai, Hagali, Salema, Lazaro and Siti in front of the family house. Immediately after arrival, Siti rushed to his mother and commented that the old man walks straight without a walking stick! After a drink and a snack, Runyoro, then a research student at the University left to go to his flat while the three visitors were resting and talking about their travel including the opening of the presents that they brought. The presents included some carvings, dresses, *'sime'* a Masai tribe's weapon similar to a machete, worn as a protection while in the bush and a spear. On that day Dorisi's family increased from five to eight. She managed to cook all the foods needed with dignity and remarkable efficiency, making life in the house happy and welcoming. The four weeks of Salema's visit included various visits in Birmingham, London, Leeds, and Llandudno. In Birmingham a notable place Salema visited was Aston University where Touwa, his son had done his BSc in Pharmacy and a PhD in Pharmaceutical Sciences. He was pleased to accompany his son to his work at his Pharmacy shop that he managed for five years. Salema spent the four weeks by touring in the day and having a drink in the evening with his family. His travel to Leeds to visit Anastasia and Jonii reassured Salema that his son was not alone in UK as he had friends who he could trust. The last day of holiday was a party, a dance and a massive barbeque at the house. Present were all the family, Dr Klemperer, Professor Wibberley, (Touwa's former tutors at the University)lots of East African students from Birmingham University. The five girls who helped Touwa during Sesilia's wedding, Asha, Sewe, Sara, Halima and Mangeni were present. The same girls made Salema's holiday a memorable occasion. Those girls cooked food for Salema and took him to numerous places in Birmingham University and the city. They also had facilitated the meeting of an array of people from many countries who were their friends and were invited to the party. After eating and drinking, Asata, a family friend and Owen's mother, responded to the music by starting to dance on the lawn. Many of the guests joined in the dancing. Everyone applauded in approval when Dr Klemperer asked Salema to dance. The party became alive and raucous and continued till one in the night.

Salema left England happy, having seen and visited his son's place of study, Aston University. On the way to the airport, Salema, Kimwai and Lazaro confirmed their satisfaction of the visit that made them very happy. The happiness led him to utter some famous words:

'When I die, it is only my feet that die, my head lives on'.

As he sat quietly in the car, reflecting on the whole travel, Salema confided to his son that he was sorry for the initial refusal to accept the invitation because he felt as if he was travelling like a bag of maize whose eyes and ears were Lazaro and the companionship of Kimwai and he wanted not to be a burden. He added that he was no longer worried about travelling and even took the opportunity to invite his hosts Dorisi, Anastasia, Jonii and George to visit him in Africa and that Touwa had to arrange the travel. With a mutual agreement Salema boarded the direct flight of British airways bound for Nairobi.

The Arrival of grandchildren:

The years passed fast as life was busy with the aspiration of making more and more money. One day Dorisi told Touwa: *'your little girl is no longer little'* that was like a surprise to Touwa who then realised that they had a teenage daughter. Teenage children can sometimes present with new growing up problems and sometimes heart break incidents that were hard to solve, and the pain due to constant arguments that could result from insignificant issues. Initially, the grief, the unpleasant atmosphere, the arguments, the disobedience and sometimes insults were unbearable to the two hard working parents. They solved problems as best as they could as there was no book of instructions to follow. Touwa was well educated with a Doctorate degree, but the teenage problems were above his ability to solve or even understand. He noted parent-hood that was the smooth and cool activities of food buying and preparation and eating together, the buying of school uniforms, watching telly programmes together, making jokes, and even going to trips together had changed. That changed suddenly to harsh moments of stunts of stubborn events at home and school, visits to school to resolve conflicts, heated arguments at home for non attendance to school. Viciousness in actions or looks, with bitterly spoken words and the inability to make sense of arguments with the unwillingness to compromise made parents worried sensing failure in their part. At one time they portioned blame to working for long hours. The children's issues and working regularly were hard for the parents, Touwa and Dorisi. They were determined to succeed as failure was not an option but pinned their faith in the hope that the rebellious nature of the teenage years would come to pass. It was during the college years that one early morning, angry parents who had not seen their daughter for months were awakened by a young man who was very polite, but shyly delivering news of the birth of a baby boy by Mkasu. It was Monday the 23rd May 1994, the date that Dorisi and Touwa woke up as grandparents. That was how grandchildren started to arrive!

The Grandchildren, the list as they came:

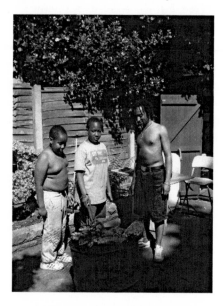

Barbeque after shed cleaning

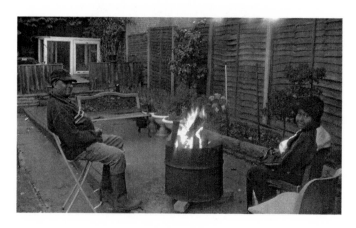

Kai & g'dad

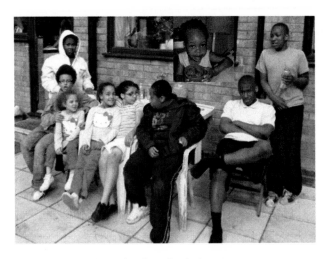

Grands after shed cleaning

The name	Time & Date of birth	Parent	Parent time of birth
Junaide Bowers (Juju)	Monday 02.00 hour 23rdMay 1994	Mkasu (Heidi Mroso)	Saturday 29th November 1975 00.02 hours
Kiambu Mroso (Big man)	Monday 22.06 hours 22nd September 1997	Hagali (Anthony Mroso)	Saturday 27th August 1977 14.28 hours
Unaysaah Mc Dowell (Nacey—petal)	Friday 04. 00 hours. 14th May 1999	Mkasu (Heidi Mroso)	Saturday 29th November 1975 00.02 hours
Kai Mroso (Kai Kai)	Monday 01.26hours 27th February 2001	Hagaly	Saturday 27th August 1977 14.28 hours

Ammarah Hector (Mara—Flower)	Thursday 14.00 hours 1st March 2001	Mkasu (Heidi Mroso)	Saturday 29th November 1975 00.02 hours
Rayyaan Hector (Ray ray)	Friday 16.00 hours 17th May 2002	Mkasu (Heidi Mroso)	Saturday 29th November 1975 00.02 hours
Renee Mroso (Princess)	Monday 20.16 hours 1st January 2007	Siti (Steven Mroso)	Sunday 13th February 1983 21.16 hours
Rowan Mroso	Sunday 03.00 hours 19th September 2010	Hagali (Anthony Mroso)	Saturday 27th August 1977 14.28 hours

Holiday to Salema's Africa:

A year of preparation was needed to embark on an African tour that was centred on visiting Salema. First, Touwa and his cousin Lazaro planned transport for 10-12 people from airport to all places planned. Second, was the making of the

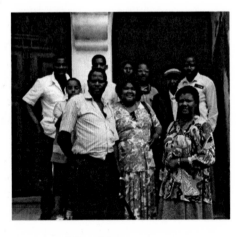

The africa tour team

timetable to name places, persons, dates and finally to confirm the travelling team. Advice on travel requirements such as clothing, to match the diverse conditions that were anticipated during the tour were also put in writing. Touwa, Dorisi, Anastasia, Jonii, Siti, Owen and Tim became the final choice of the team that was to travel to Africa to visit Salema. A timetable of travel showed the extent of driving, sleeping and pleasure times. Finances were planned to cover eventualities. One request that surprised everyone was the need of a rain cover and jumper or coat for the cold areas. That request was ignored as no one expected Africa to be cold. *'The African Safari travel timetable of July 1994'* was a detailed account of dates, times, places and individuals to meet. The Sabena Belgian Airlines left London to Brussels to Entebbe in Uganda and finally to Nairobi Kenya. At the airport on arrival cousin Lazaro and Touwa's brother Tabu, were at hand to take the group to Touwa's cousin, Margaret Katondo's house in Nairobi for a freshening in order to travel to Eldoret to meet Dorisi's cousin, Dr. Gosnell York who was teaching at the University. The travel to Eldoret was the first test of the true climate of Africa witnessed by those in the team that had never visited the continent and even it was also a surprise to the Africans. The team left the sunny and warm weather in Nairobi, just south of the Equator, travelling north-westwards for a planned four hour journey. The first obstacle was a rough road forcing Minja, the driver of the mini bus, to go at slower speeds. The second obstacle was the poor road markings making it difficult to locate the destination, a whole University. The third was not an obstacle but a problem. As the team was crossing the equator from then south to north, there was a sign that alerted travellers when they crossed the Equator, but it could not be seen due to heavy fog and it was exceedingly cold. All the warm attire was left at Katondo's house in Nairobi as Eldoret travel was only an overnight stay. The minibus was not well closed to protect the passengers from the cold. Cousin Lazaro a seasoned traveller and brother Tabu could have anticipated the cold so he produced a bottle of 'konyagi' the local alcoholic spirit drink! The kids Siti and his friend Owen, (*Owen, was a friend of Siti, is seen on picture above with Tim, Jonii and Anastasia*)were enjoying their soft drinks. All the adults in the bus welcomed Lazaro's offer by drinking slowly on a rota basis. When it came to give to Dorisi the b o t t l e , Touwa said to Lazaro that she does not drink. It was so cold that Dorisi wanted a little drink,

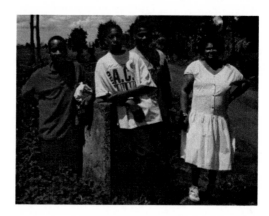

Visitors at Salemas

so she shouted: *'gi'me some no!'* meaning *'give me the drink now!'* Everyone was surprised to see Dorisi drinking, an act signifying how cold it was when the team travelled to Eldoret. It was midnight when Dr York was awakened by Dorisi calling. He was happy to see her, although she was expected to arrive much earlier as per timetable. The half day was spent by visiting friends like Dr Sewe at Moi University and the town of Eldoret prior to returning to Nairobi. The next day, Tabu left the team as he had to go to Mwingi where he was a teacher. The team followed a long dusty road to Loitokitok, Lasit, and to Salema's boundary farm. Pictured are Salema and Siti on the day the team arrived at the boundary farm. The welcome was majestic. Waiting for the team were: 'm*zee*' Salema (the title of '*mzee*' which means old man, was an African way of respect), Ndesumbuka, Melikoi, with his wife Raheli and all other 22 children of mzee Salema, Fr. Phillipo (*a friend of Ndesumbuka*) and all the neighbours. The party started in earnest with '*mbege*' the local brew being shared so freely as if it would never finish. Large pieces of roast meat were presented to the guests. The brothers Ndesumbuka, Melikoi, Tabu and Tabuni, stayed with the guests

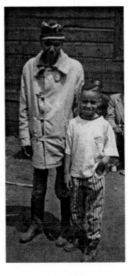

Siti visit to Nanjara

guiding them to all that was happening. Touwa and Lazaro

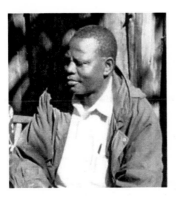

Cousin Lazaro

were the leaders in the tours, were seated quietly planning, and checking the next phase of the timetable. The driver Minja, was always had the vehicle ready for the next move as per instructions from Lazaro. Every day for seven days the team enjoyed a grand party in the village of Nanjara and Tarakea. Invitations were done by a sister, a brother or an uncle.

There were times when mzee Salema had to make the choice for the party as there were more offers than time would allow. A farewell party was at uncle Kimwai who had accompanied Salema to the UK tour. It was a grand occasion the started with drinks, roasting, dancing and eventually school children performing songs and poems.

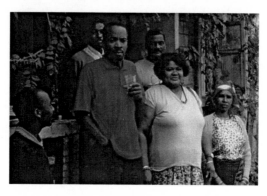

Visitors and hosts at Nanjara2

Safari park adventures:

After seven days of drinking, eating, resting with no worries, no phone calls, no bad news, it was no wonder everyone increased in weight and the space in the mini van appeared inadequate for the same number of passengers who experienced being tightly packed. From Nanjara the team travelled to Moshi town then to Arusha where preparations to go to Manyara and then to Ngorongoro Crater National park were made. The dusty roads, the mighty distances, the road side businesses, the parks, the scenery and finally the array of animals were all experienced in a breath-taking 5 day non-stop tour. The return journey included a stop at Arusha for resting and socializing with friends of Touwa like

Kishe and Ngaleku. It was at a party hoisted on the lawn at Kishe's house, when the cool day temperatures dropped as the evening approached. It was such a cold evening reminding everyone that Africa can be cold. The funny part of this occasion was that everyone had left the warm clothing at the hotel, hence experiencing the full African chill. Help however was at hand when Kishe's wife offered the guests 'kanga' (*an African sheet like decorated material usually worn as a loin cloth*)to cover and offset the effects of the cold air.

It took the whole day travelling from Arusha to Dar es Salaam a 600km distance. Touwa was leading the way to Mbezi where he had built his house years earlier but when he reached there he did not recognize it and asked the driver to go further. After a short drive that was two or three kilometres, Dorisi saw a road sign that she was sure it meant they had passed Mbezi. They all agreed to go back and by sheer chance stopped near a pub. The family in Mbezi consisting of Ndesumbuka, Melikoi, Tarimo and Bavo and an array of close friends saw the team first and started calling. Touwa was relieved to hear his brother calling as he new he was home, and the whole group had a drink and a rest in the warm coastal air of Dar es Salaam. The Dar es Salaam tour included shopping, visiting friends with whom food and drinks became the welcoming site. A trip to Zanzibar and Bagamoyo to see the relics that depicted the horrors of slavery could have concluded the 6 day stay in Dar es Salaam but for the surprise planned by Runyoro that changed the well followed timetable. Runyoro was a friend of Touwa, previously in Birmingham and played a vital work in taking Salema around the city during his Birmingham visit.

The Dar es Salaam wedding:

A fast boat took the travelling team on an early morning trip to Zanzibar Island, with a return ticket in the afternoon. On arrival at the water front, Runyoro's friends met the travelling team to spring up a surprise. The team was directed to a church, it was to witness a marriage oath ceremony at St Joseph church. The big surprise was that it was Touwa's friend Runyoro who was getting married to a beautiful girl named Martha. The long, slow, colourful and above all very pleasant singing ceremony came to an end after an hour and a half, followed by the trip to

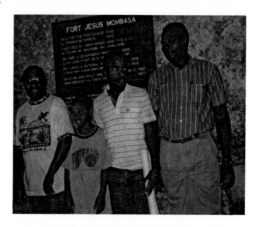

With Lazaro in Mombasa

the reception. At the reception, the bride and groom was welcome to the hall by a live band that sang many foot tapping songs reciting the bride and grooms names. The beer and food that followed was as abundant as the beautiful girls dressed in bridesmaids' attire and serving everyone in the hall. The dancing, the eating and drinking after the numerous witty speeches, continued without the realisation that it was midnight. Shaking hands and hugs, Touwa and his travelling team said bye-bye to the married couple and sped to Mbezi for a short sleep. The travelling, the drinking and lack of rest, was the reason everyone was tired and needed a day of recuperation, a very odd concept as the team was on a holiday! The rest day allowed reflecting, that led to a decision to have a party to say thanks to all who made the stay memorable. Dorisi and Anastasia would cook, Touwa, Tim and Jonii would organize the drinks, while Ndesumbuka and Melikoi would do the invitations. The boys who were just eleven were encouraged to visit the friends they had made and relax. At Melikoi's house the women embarked on the cooking using charcoal and wood in place of gas or electricity. By six in the evening the guests were arriving and the party of drinking, music and food started. Speeches of thanking and good bye dominated the evening that continued to the early hours of the morning. With or without hangover, the team had to start the outbound journey to Tanga. That time the team included one more person and that was Salema.

From Dar es Salaam with glee:

The journey from Dar es Salaam to Tanga and onwards to Mombasa and Nairobi was full of reflections on the friends made, the sites seen, the enjoyment derived from the warm welcome received and the array of gifts that were given. The African safari was coming to an end; the memory would be through the photographs taken. A subdued moment during the few hours of travel occurred as a result of the travellers reflecting on friends they had left behind. The travel was comfortable and relaxing as the team could stop to buy fresh fruits at road side stalls, Siti could have a chat with his granddad and Lazaro could continue giving a commentary on places passed. At Tanga town, Touwa took the opportunity of showing his dad and friends, Usagara Secondary School, the high school he attended. The journey continued to Mombasa and Malindi where tourist sites were visited. On the Indian Ocean beach at Mombasa, the team observed a very low tide, when people could walk far into the sea to find shells. It was at that time Salema's paternal instincts were apparent, such that he made Lazaro run to the sea to call Dorisi and Touwa who had wandered a bit too far to cause concern. On seeing the couple coming back Salema smiled, making Dorisi to comment: *'Your dad thinks you are still a kid'.* The day at the beach while eating peppered roast cassava, coconut water and tasting of *'halua'*(exceedingly sweet jelly strings)and finally a cool beer, made an end to a smooth day on the beach, enabling the team to start the travel to Nairobi.

From Mombasa to Nairobi the team passed through Tsavo National Park that was made famous by a book: *'Simba wa Tsavo'* (*Swahili for The lion of Tsavo*). That book was about a lion that acquired a taste for human flesh. The lion avoided capture and it became so cunning that it could take and devour at will the Indian railway labourers. The bravery and the cunning nature of the lion was that it picked humans from inside the extra protected tents and within minutes sped into the bush eat the victim and game wardens with rifles could not see it to shoot. The remains of the victims were found but never the lion until the near completion of the railway.

At Nairobi, Mr and Mrs Katondo, arranged a meal at *'Bomas of Kenya'*, a place where food meant meat. The meat however was eaten is style, as each source of meat had its own sauce. There was the usual beef, lamb, chicken and pork. The surprise to all, except Katondo was the new sources of meat like wilder beast, giraffe, buffalo, Zebra, ostrich, impala and surprisingly that of crocodile. Salema and Anastasia with the boys gave thumbs down to crocodile. Touwa, Lazaro, Dorisi Jonii and Tim said they would try. For the team it was the first time they saw crocodile meat let alone tasting it. After tasting, someone said: *'could I have some more?'* it prompted everyone to taste or eat crocodile meat. The meal was a success as the team emerged from the restaurant well fed having eaten and liked crocodile and other exotic animals' meat. The next day it was planned to visit Touwa's brother Tabu, who was a teacher in Mwingi Secondary school.

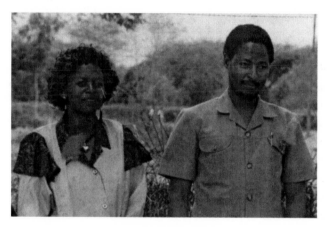

Tabu & Kavengi

At Tabu's residence, Kavengi, his wife with her beautiful smile greeted all the team members before offering a drink which was a start of a feast. As that region was dry, Tabu was proud to show his father how they harvested rain water to boost the meagre water supply. Looking at the area and noticing how arid it was, Touwa could not resist asking his brother why he chose to go so far to the dry region. Before Tabu could answer Salema interrupted and drew the attention to Touwa to check who was closer to home. That visit at Mwingi was concluded happily with Tabu joining the team to Nairobi for the farewell at the airport the next day. The journey to Nairobi airport was a sad affair as there were too many good byes to friends and family and the many happy moments logged in the memory. In the morning the preparations to the airport were in time and Minja, the driver was probably looking forward for a well earned rest after clocking nearly 3000 Km drive to various short and long trips in Kenya and Tanzania. He started the engine and slowly moved towards the airport. It was after one or two kilometres drive away when the gearbox caught fire. A quick exit and use of extinguisher saved all. The cause was that the oil was suddenly lost as the rusted bolt the covers the engine fell off, making the hot oil flow out profusely. That incident forced hasty good-byes from Touwa, Dorisi, Anastasia, Jonii, Tim, Siti and Owen to Salema, Lazaro, Tabu and Minja who were left with the broken down mini-van that had served so faithfully for the past 20 days.

The story of Salema's Africa was narrated to many friends who longed to visit Africa one day. When Jonii was telling friends about his travels, he never forgot to tell when a bird stole his sandwich to feed it partner (a bird) up in the tree, a true happening that occurred at Manyara National park. With the laugh and excitement the stories of the African trip were told and retold as the years sped by. Life in Birmingham and Leeds, for the families of Touwa and Jonii continued with the usual *'glee and tears, the ups and downs of life, as the years speed by'.*

Melikoi's visit to Birmingham:

The visit to Africa was a success; friendships that were made led to communications and eventually invitations. Melikoi's wife, Raheli was instrumental in the planning and supply of dinners for the travellers in Nanjara and in Dar es Salaam. Raheli was a softly spoken and well-mannered intelligent woman, who accompanied by her husband Melikoi on the visit to Birmingham to reciprocate the hospitality. The good aspect of the visit was that it was both a family visit and a country tour as there were other friends apart from his brother that they could visit. The two brothers took the opportunity to

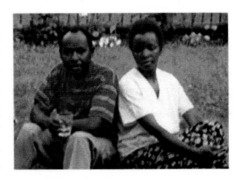

Melikoi and Raheli in brum

know each other better by recalling their experiences during the periods they were apart.

Melikoi, Touwa's younger brother was the next after Ndesumbuka, smaller in stature and darker in skin complexion than the other brothers had basic primary education that he advanced by continuous learning. His travel to England was also an opportunity to expand his knowledge by visiting some engineering workshops to see the level of work performed. The trust and friendship of the two brothers was mutual because Melikoi helped in the completion of Mbezi house project. Melikoi pleased all brothers by ensuring that Salema's first visit to Mbezi was as homely as possible by preparing *'mbege'* for that occasion. The presence of Melikoi in Mbezi attracted Ndesumbuka to stay there after his studies in Russia. Ndesumbuka like many of the Nanjara born group that was working in Dar es Salaam made Mbezi as their permanent home. The large Nanjara community in Mbezi owes that presence to Melikoi who was their first resident. In their conversations Melikoi revealed to Touwa that after finishing his primary education, he could not proceed as Ndesumbuka and Tabu. Salema tried but in vein to send him for more studies due to lack of funds. He could not afford to help him that time due to complex home problems and cash that was essential to fund school fees. Melikoi left home for Arusha to work in a textile factory, while involved in a correspondence school that he too failed to complete due to finances as his salary then could not cover such extra costs. He left Arusha to Dar es Salaam to join his brother who sent him to a vocational school that helped him to get better jobs and that was a start of a better independent living. After marriage and further studies he gained a certificate of *'Precision Machining'*. Melikoi was a trained draftsman, good at tool making and a brilliant innovator. He showed interest in visiting some tool making engineering workshops to brighten his horizons in addition to enjoying British tour sites. Raheli a quietly spoken woman enjoyed shopping trips with Dorisi in Birmingham and with Anastasia in Leeds. A trip to Llandudno and the great sight seeing that the trip involved concluded their four week stay. It was in the year that the first grandson, Junaide, became a year old. The years that followed, there were the arrival of Kiambu and Unaysaah who welcomed the year 2000 when there were many predicted unforeseen disasters such as computer crashes.

Meeting with Flora:

In June 1999, Touwa had travelled to Tanzania the homeland to visit his father and all his relatives. Dorisi was in a West midland bus on her way home after a staff meeting at Solihull Hospital. It was when she heard some girls conversing in Swahili, Touwa's national language. She took the opportunity to greet the girls *'jambo'* meaning hello in Swahili. The girls were surprised to realise their conversation was overheard. Flora, a talkative pregnant girl, started to converse in Swahili with Dorisi to find out that she knew only a few words of the language. From their introductions, it was then realised that Flora was from Tanzania and she was soon going to Heartlands hospital to have the baby. To the surprise of Flora, Dorisi revealed that she worked at that hospital and that her husband was Tanzanian as Flora. Flora was a student with plans to get married before the birth of the child. It was a surprise to Dorisi who did not expect an invite but instead, she was asked to help in organizing the wedding for Flora! Dorisi replied calmly, *'I shall tell my husband on arrival and you will be informed'.* With those words, they parted to ponder on the significance of the request. Touwa was glad to be given such an honour, made plans to meet Flora, and eventually Allesandro, the husband to be; and plans for the wedding started. Wedding rings, food and drinks supply, plans to decorate the hall, hair styles plans and numerous other wedding tasks were achieved using friends like Ellie and Monica (Ellie's sister)who prepared foods, Anastasia(Dorisi's Sister)who made the cake. The success of the wedding was measured by the happiness of all the guests who ate and drank at the hotel reception that continued till the hours of the morning at Flora's flat. After the birth of Paulo, the couple moved to

Italy. A year later a passionate request by phone, was to attend a church wedding for Flora and Allesandro. Dorisi and Touwa flew to Milan and eventually drive to Triviglio, Ellie, Monica and her daughters drove their camper to Triviglio Allesandro's home. The group from Birmingham met one from Tanzania that included Flora's mum, auntie, two sisters and a priest Mapunda joining the hosts that was Flora, Paulo and Allesandro. In a three floor apartment there also were a sister and two brothers, including the parents of Allesandro. The wedding conducted in Italian and in. Swahili was a surprise to many Italians but not as much as when in the

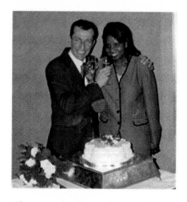

Flora and allesandro wedding

evening the African drums started to sound from the Ferri family estate unlike any other Italian wedding. The friendship of the two families of Touwa and Allesandro did not end there as ten years later (2009)an invite to go back to Triviglio for a double celebration was honoured. The first was the confirmation of Paulo and the week later was the ordination of Kessy, (a Tanzanian)to priesthood.

Paulo's confirmation was a big celebration when all ten year olds are confirmed into the Church and each family have a celebration. The family celebration at Ferri's estate (Allesandro's home)started at one in the afternoon. It was a nine course lunch that continued to be a supper and with drinks and music, it could be one of the best meals in the world.

The week that followed, Touwa and Dorisi took another flight to Triviglio to attend the church service and eventual celebration at the seminary that marked the ordination of several

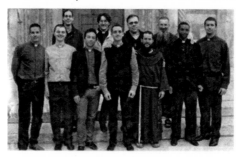

Priest with Kessy

priests from many parts of the world including Rev. Baltazary Kessy at San Zeno Cathedral in Verona. (Picture by the Verona fedele of 24 May 2009). The attendance of the ordination was rewarded with a day boat trip in Venice. The spectacular beauty of the city became a treasured memory for Dorisi and Touwa.

The visit of Flora, Allesandro and Paulo a year later, to Dorisi and Touwa in Birmingham made the already good friendship an everlasting one.

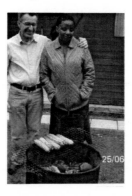

A barbeque at brum

CHAPTER 10

Dorisi and Touwa;
Life in the Millennium

The millennium and the doom predictions:

As the year 2000 approached, there were lots of comments on the happenings that would occur, some religious, some technical, while the many predictions of disasters could not pass without being noticed or cause some worry. The computer outage predictions were the most costly but proved to be false. Lots of money was exchanged for updates, warning leaflets and even the government set up a crisis body to oversee the anticipated problems. As the UK watched, Japanese, Chinese and Australian entry into the millennium, the fireworks continued as usual the stock exchange was functioning and the computers were properly functioning. Many people were let down financially by the doomsday predictions that prompted people to carry on expensive computer updates.

All that came to pass without incidents.

Bonding with grandchildren:

In the year 2000, Touwa and his wife Dorisi were happy, healthy, with enough but not wealthy and definitely wise. They had seen and experienced the worries, the tears and the disappointments brought about during teenage years of their then teenage children. There were also some happy moments when the children made progress and were getting ahead in life. They were mentally strong to guide their children towards independent living and into their desired careers. The grandchildren as they came with the happiness they radiated to the family start to mellow and soften the previously strict Dorisi and Touwa into soft, protective and loving grandparents. As the children were leaving home one by one, the unique bonds between grandparents and grandchildren were very strong fuelled by an array of social events. The barbeques with the young grandchildren became a social event triggered by any excuse.

There arose:

- *a planting season party,*
- *a pond cleaning party,*
- *a shed tidying party,*
- *a potato harvesting party*
- *a January-June Birthdays party,*
- *a July—December Birthdays party*

The big list of bonding periods with the grandchildren influenced a friend to comment on Touwa and Dorisi as *"the happiest grandparents in the world"*. The two grandparents enhanced such happiness in their quest for life by travelling whenever an opportunity arose. It was during the travelling years that the children of Touwa and Dorisi were having the talk of shouldering the growing pains of their own children, adding to the task of being grandparents to being mentors and advisers to their children. The characters of the then grown up children were manifested. The observed characters could be shaped by life numerous demands and influence of friends and possibly finances. The resultant portrayed adult description could include those who were reliable, loving and cared for the family and those who had an inward looking in life and cared little of others. It was with satisfaction that the path the children chose led them to a good level independence and the ability to stand on their own feet and basically contented.

The list below will act a brief travel monologue:

Year	Activity	Country & Places visited with comments
1981	Touwa & Dorisi visit to Russia to visit Ndesumbuka	USSR Moscow & Zaporozhye First time in a communist state
1990	Touwa, Mkasu, Hagali and Siti visits St Kitts in West Indies	Touwa's first Meeting with Peter York, Dorisi's Dad Dorisi did a surprise when she turned up in St. Kitts at that time
1992	Salema Visits UK accompanied by Moshi and uncle Kimwai	A 4-week tour. Birmingham, Leeds. Llandudno. Rhyl. A big barbeque and dance party
1992	Weekend cruise to Denmark	Sailing in the north sea first experience in sea travel
1993	Mediterranean Cruise	Italy Egypt, Israel, Greece and Turkey Experienced rough seas

1994	Family Group travel to Tanzania	Kenya: Mombasa, Nairobi, Tanzania: Dar, Manyara, Ngorongoro, Arusha, Moshi, Nanjara Tarakea & Lasit and Zanzibar by fast boat A surprise wedding of Runyoro in Dar and a taste of crocodile meat Touwa, Dorisi, Anastasia,(Anna)Jonii (,Levi,)Tim, (Loxley Wright), Siti (Steven)& Owen
1995	Melikoi & Raheli visit Birmingham	Visit of London Leeds, Llandudno and various sites in Birmingham Melikoi enjoyment of motorway drive Party and barbeques
1998	South American Cruise by Touwa and Dorisi	21 day cruise to Brazil(Sao Paulo), Rio de Janeiro, Recife, Salvador, Senegal (Dakar), Tenerife, Morocco(Casablanca & Marrakech and in Ali Baba Market, Andalusia, Barcelona and back to Italy(Genoa)Coldest period as crossing the equator, salt mines in Senegal
1999	Dorisi trip to Tanzania and ST Kitts	To Tanzania with Donita and Kiambu visit Mikumi national park Trip to St Kitts was due to the death of her father Peter York that occurred after Tanzania trip was made
2000	Touwa and Dorisi to Italy to Flora's wedding,	Visit Milan, and Malpensa & Travegglio Floras relatives from Tanzania and Europe were in the wedding A good wedding plenty to eat and drink met priests and a Bishop from Tanzania

2002	Touwa travel & Dorisi to Las Vegas	Arranged by Winston Brown, visits to Arizona and California and the great canyon First time in America later in that year visit to Tanzania for Touwa's Dad's funeral
2003	Dorisi & Touwa Caribbean Cruise	Visits to Kissime, St Thomas, St John, Dominican Republic, Bahamas Dorisi meet her primary school teacher Ronald
2004	Ndesumbuka and his wife Simforosa visits Touwa in Birmingham	Visit London, The Thames cruise, Llandudno, Leeds and Birmingham sites Rekindled his previous visits and baby sitting duties as a student in USSR
2005	Touwa and Dorisi visits St Louis in USA	St Louise, Martin Luther King historical places, Slavery trail. Elvis Priestly story in Memphis A number of museums dedicated to reviving the historical places
2006	Holiday in Tenerife	Sun, sand and Sangria
2007	Holiday to Cyprus	Travel to historical sites Noted the line of division of Cyprus a joke about ABC(another b* * * church, cathedral or castle)
2007	Holliday to Thailand	All about the Buddha
2008	Holiday to Hawaii	Fly to Chicago, then another flight to Seattle, drive to Vancouver in Canada for the cruise start to Hawaii Volcanoes that form no mountains
2009	Touwa and Dorisi Cruise to Panama and Central America	Flight to Florida, cruise to Panama, Belize, Costa Rica The Panama Canal, Pineapple cultivation and export venture in Costa Rica and coffee

2010	Cuba visit Holliday first visit	Havana and Sugar factory that was defunct (Hotel: The Blau in Varadero) Had a chance to drive a steam train
2011	Cuba Visit holiday second visit	Varadero (Meli las Americas)and in Havana (Melia Havana)visited Bay of Pigs, Central Cuba (Trinidad)Santa Clara and valley of Vinales in Western Cuba show Tropicana was a theatre experience

When Salema was eighty one:

The millennium and the fears that were rumoured passed; holidays and travelling plans were made. In a small pub, the Shaftmoor, Touwa and many of the punters welcome the year 2002 as the clock struck midnight. *"Happy new year and all the best the year would bring"* was what was heard or spoken by everyone in the pub. As usual holiday plans for that year were made.

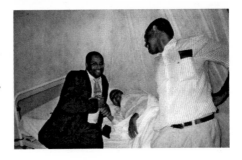

When Salema was ill

It was one phone call, by Touwa's friend Mwajuma, who reported that Salema was in hospital where he needed oxygen. Within two hours Touwa made a call to Ndesumbuka asking him to collect him and Dorisi the next day in the evening at Dar es Salaam airport. The speed in getting a ticket that fast was a pleasant surprise to both brothers who were mutually happy. It was a short drive from the airport to Salema's hospital bed. It was when Salema opened his eyes to see Dorisi that he smiled and realised she had travelled far to see him. When Salema attempted to tell Touwa about the expenses incurred in that visit as unnecessary, Ndesumbuka intervened and simply said to his dad: *'It is just respect and love'*. Salema's happiness did not end there, as he strongly indicated he

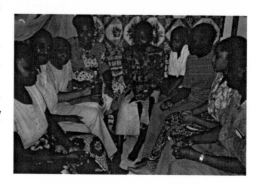

Salema with his close family

wanted to be discharged to go home. A doctor was contacted but he was of a junior rank and could not do that alone. He however said it was possible after approval from the hospital registrar. The hope was that Salema could be ready to go home the next day. In the morning, Ndesumbuka and Touwa went to the hospital to bring their father home. When that request was granted Salema was visibly happy, talking, laughing, and even making jokes, although he was weak. The three week holiday, that started as an emergency became more relaxing as Salema was feeling better. Due to other travel commitments Touwa and Ndesumbuka decided to cut the holiday to two weeks by arranging for an earlier airline ticket. Several attempts to get a ticket failed so Dorisi and Touwa stayed with Salema for the full three weeks. Salema was well enough to go out and enjoy a little drink. After the three weeks, Touwa and Dorisi boarded the plane to return to UK via Amsterdam. The connection to Birmingham was eventually achieved after several changes of the Gate numbers, a problem which was not apparent at that time. On arrival at Birmingham, it was realised that

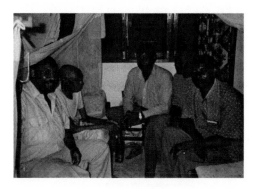

**Touwa, Salema, Tabuni,
Melikoi and Ndesumbuka**

there was a start of a strike at Amsterdam and many connecting flights were delayed for several hours or days. It was with luck that there was no delay for Touwa and Dorisi who were to travel to the USA the next day.

The travel to the United States, to Las Vegas was without problems and was an enjoyable holiday. Correspondence between Ndesumbuka and Touwa on the update of Salema's health was regular and continued after the Las Vegas holiday. One day in September at 10 am, a phone call with the fewest words was received. *'Dad has passed away'*, said the shaky voice of Ndesumbuka, who also received a very short answer: *'ok I understand'* and immediately switched off the phone as Touwa burst into tears of sorrow and crying. After half an hour Touwa made a call to his brother to say that he would travel as soon as an airline ticket was secured.

It was such luck that a single attempt to get a ticket for the next day was obtained. On arrival at Dar es Salaam, Touwa was collected by Ndesumbuka's friend Nyichomba, and driven to the family house to meet the house full of mourners. The crying, the sorrow, the sad faces he saw were too much for Touwa to avoid crying again. There was no sleeping that night; it was for talking and comforting each other among the family and friends The next morning funeral timetable started and Touwa's task was to ensure collection of the body of Salema from the mortuary where he had to supervise the dressing up and finally placing the body in the coffin. Touwa was very stressed such that he had to be helped to fix the neck tie to fit on his father's body. With the coffin closed Touwa placed a hibiscus flower on it as the journey to the family house where a funeral ceremony was to start. It was after that ceremony that the journey to the burial site was started. It took a whole night of travelling in two coaches and some cars for the almost 600km to Nanjara, Salema's birth place. Salema was laid to rest into a grave next to that of Mkasu, his first wife. It was September, 13th, 2002, forty three years since Mkasu died. Salema's family was then consisting of 22 children, 13 boys and 9 girls, one boy was adopted, 145 grandchildren and over 50 great grandchildren. There were some great-great grand children.

Ndesumbuka's visit to Birmingham:

Life in general was subdued after the passing of Salema for a period of one year when a great memorial to celebrate Salema's life was conducted by all his family members. (83) The memorial celebrations were awash with plenty of *'mbege'* drinking, meat eating, chatting and laughter. The influence of 'mbege' would induce the singing and possibly dancing to remember him for what he used to provide to others. That was the time he was remembered for his wisdom, wit, kindness, loving and a hard worker and faithful to his three wives as it was known that he had no other children outside the three relationships. The 22 children were living in good harmony, as Salema had ensured wealth distribution when he was alive to the satisfaction of all. Those who did not have a piece of land were given, in addition those who had lands of their own like Touwa, Ndesumbuka, Melikoi and Tabuni were given a plot for use as if needed as a place of final rest. It was in one of the visits that Touwa was shown the land his father had given him. In turn he asked one of the brothers, the adopted one, Mashaka to care for it. It was also during the visit that Ndesumbuka showed a desire to take his wife to UK for a tour. (84)In a mutual agreement plans were set in motion for a visit that took place in the summer of 2004. To ask to tour a rich country like Britain from a poor country like Tanzania, there were hurdles to overcome in addition to passports and visas. The extra hurdles included a proof that one would return home, a financial check to support oneself and even the check of the financial position of the parson to be visited. Ndesumbuka and Simforosa did overcome the hurdles and visited Touwa in Birmingham. For Ndesumbuka, Birmingham was well known to him from the days of his studies in USSR, when he made frequent summer holiday visits to see his brother. For Simforosa it was the first time of going outside Tanzania. The tour was planned to give Simforosa a good exposure of the country and ensure a great enjoyment. The two plans were accomplished by visiting Birmingham city, travel to Leeds, to London and a Thames river cruise and to see Buckingham Palace and finally a trip to Wales in Llandudno and Rhyl. The social life included barbeques, theatre, pub and restaurant visits. Ndesumbuka was glad to see the baby he used to baby-sit, Siti, who had become a big boy, then aged 21. The tour helped to cement the bond of the two brothers who were facing life after Salema.

Life with grandchildren:

The arrival of grandchildren is a shock to many a man or woman as it becomes a real reminder that one is getting older, but the shock is superseded by the joy they bring to one's quality of life. When very young, grandchildren hug and hold to grandparents so loving that there is no comparison. As they grow a bit, they portray their parents good, bad and funny habits, that is seen by grandparents. When they portray wit, give laughter, the absolute willingness to help, learn and participate in stories no matter how many times they hear, or watch films numerous times, make grandchildren excellent companions for grandparents. The eagerness to show things they know, sometimes to share secrets that they would not tell their parents, makes being a grandparent a pleasure. If you record a conversation of a group of grandparents they talk about their grandchildren with pride, and in fact there is a hidden competition to tell the most hilarious story of an incident with ones grandchild. The great moments of counting 1 to 10 and the alphabet a, b, c . . . and later the school songs of a, b, c, d e, f g . . . are never completed until heard and congratulated by a grandparent. Touwa in year 2011, with his eight grandchildren, found all the joy grandchildren can give and they all enjoy to sing the famous song: *'haya o haya haya hee'* and the only story he knew was about *'Kalumekenge'.*

The first decade of the millennium was gone as the coming of the New Year 2011 was celebrated as usual. The wish for good health, wealth and possibly wisdom may be granted in many ways. Some may be well, some ill, some make money and some loose, but at the end of the year, there is the need to thank the Lord and welcome the next year.

The surgical operation of Touwa in 2011 was the reason he was celebrating the coming of the New Year 2012. In appreciation to all who looked after him in hospital he wrote:

The poem after surgery:

Me and my Blood Pressure

(A tribute to the consultant Mr Pracy and his Team, the ward 408 staff who cared for me before during and after the thyroidectomy)

It was the first time; I was in a consultation for a pre-operation
It was also the first time that I discussed my own operation.
My health status was checked, to enable a safe operation,
Despite being reassured, my blood pressure was racing to high

Meeting the consultant was pleasing and reassuring,
He checked by feeling the neck swelling while reassuring
As the staff before him, the best was his reassuring; my blood pressure was not so high.

On the operation day, my son Steven drove us fast,
To be there on time, after a whole night of fast
'Nil by mouth' was the order; I had to abide by that fast
While waiting to be called, my blood pressure was high

When I was called first, I stood to attention,
To measure my blood pressure was the action,
Her calmness did not help much in my reaction
As the instrument showed, my pressure was high

A member in Mr Pracy's team called, it was for a review in preparation,
She gave me stockings to prevent DVT, this was a precaution
Her reassurance matched her thorough checks of information,
The process was understood and my blood pressure was not so high

The surgeon in Mr Pracy's team called, it was to detail on the operation
He radiated intelligence and confidence, that was calming in an operation
He reviewed the notes, marked the area to make the cut in the operation,
'*The problem is small*', he said and my blood pressure was not so high

The anaesthetist in Mr Pracy's team called, it was to explain anaesthesia
He checked the neck, the airways while talking about anaesthesia
He made me laugh and dispelled any worries associated with anaesthesia.
'*The next call was to theatre*', he said, and my blood pressure was not so high

The pre-op sitting started and finally only two people were left to wait,
'*The unit closes at two thirty p.m.*' said the nurse, sensing an extra wait.
Reassuringly she added, '*ward 408 was the place to go to wait*'
The slight change of plans was minor but my blood pressure was on the high

With a theatre gown and DVT white stockings worn, it was off to ward 408 walking
In any other place, it would look comic, but here, without glance they kept walking
Arriving with the theatre attendant at ward 408 reception ended the walking
With others we waited, some sad, crying or praying, the blood pressure shot high

At about three p.m. I was called, walked to the theatre, where? I cannot remember
On a bed I sat, taking off all except the theatre gown. I kissed my wife to remember
I was now alone, lying down and wheeled to theatre no. 15 reception, that I remember
I thought, all should be OK; so far all was well but my blood pressure was high

The small room full of medicines & instruments with staff that was very clever
Finally he wired me to such instruments that to decipher one had to be clever
Waiting for the last patient to recover, I laid there talking to three staff of the theatre
With their genuine calming talk, I felt as good as normal but the pressure was high

'I am your anaesthetist replacing the one you saw earlier' said a voice calmly
She showed good personality, knowledge and confidence, above all she acted calmly
On the back of my right hand she placed a cannula, for the medicine of tranquillity

It was half past three, as per clock, I was drifting more into
sleep and tranquillity

In a few seconds with oxygen on my nose and mouth, I
heard many voices
It was 4 hours not seconds, opened my eyes, and then heard
'the op is done', voices
The morphine in my system made me happy and sleepy but
awoken by the voices
Next I opened the eyes I saw Dora, Anthony, Steven &
Renee as they heard my voice

After a drink of water and juices I drifted to sleep in ward
408, after the operation
No more could I say my first time, as I saw the result of a
two hour operation
A view in the mirror, the cut was like *'Frankenstein movie'*
after operation
At age sixty two, I was not suffering, and I concluded it was
a good operation

A nurse with a slight limp, walking, came to check my
health observations
She gave me good news of my family overnight seeking
observation
She was so gentle, professional and selfless in doing the
observations
I started to feel happy as if I was no longer ill based on that
observation

The surgeon came in, to check and inform on the operation
success

No complications, and anticipated nil problems in the healing process

The timetable for removal of tubes and clips was put into progress

I was so happy; I found neither a question to ask, nor a point to discuss

The next day I was on the list for discharge, and I was happy

The nurse removed some clips and the mighty tube and I was happy

She was gentle and professional, the painless process made me happy

When Dora, my wife came to take me home, I was very happy

At home as I arrived, the family was in excitement; eager to see my neck

The granddaughter voiced if they took off the head by cutting the neck

Asked if I could eat, 'Yes I said' as the cut was on the skin of the neck

She was happy, and we all laughed that all will be well with the neck

(From Dr. P V Mroso—patient for partial thyroidectomy surgery in ward 408 0n 20 & 21 /09/ 2011)

Ageing, health & wisdom:

A month after the operation, Touwa was back to health and was back to work enjoying his gardening and the usual holidays. The ill health made Touwa reflect on past event remembering those relatives and close friends who had passed away. In addition to his father Salema, it was

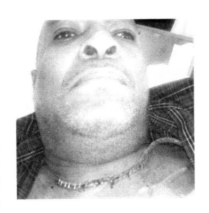

Touwa thyroid ops

uncle Mkosi, brother Salimu, childhood school friend Shirima, and cousin Lazaro. Reflections of the past influenced Touwa to think of the future but not for him but for the younger ones that was the children and grandchildren. Together, Dorisi and Touwa enjoyed the progress of the young ones and were ready to offer their combined wisdom to influence their future to prosperity.

As the years sped by the healthy living that we all take for granted when we are young starts for the majority to be interrupted with episodes of feeling unwell, periods of pain and an increase in the need for medical care. With the passing years one finds out the meaning of some medical terms that they never believed they existed as the list below may suggest.

A few days after 62, Touwa was to undergo a surgical operation to remove a swelling gland. The *partial thyroidectomy* as it was called was successful. Work and normal activities were resumed. Eight months later still aged 62 a set of events took place that was remembered and put in context as follows:

A thank you to Mr Whiting and his team, Dr Walt (CT scan)the McMillan nurses, the surgeon Prof. Alderson and his team, the nurses in recovery and in wards 302 and 727 and all other care staff who looked after me

Me and the GIST:

I was at work, healthy but not wealthy busy packing some boxes to send away for charity
When I lifted a box that was probably a bit heavy, I thought I pulled a muscle in my body
I rubbed some gel and ointments and the condition was improving so I thought nothing iffy
The week that followed I felt a feeling of hunger that was frequent and intense to give me some worry
I swallowed some antacids to alleviate the pain but in vain, such that a visit to a GP was necessary

The thorough diagnosis was done and Omeprazole was prescribed by the Doctor
The relief was achieved, happiness was attained and praise was given to the Doctor
A week later, I was in good health, an episode of fainting, made it vital to see the Doctor
The thorough check ruled out heart problems but suspicion of anaemia was noted by the Doctor

A blood test to confirm the anaemia and iron tablets were prescribed to solve the problem

It took a week to do the test but the quick results, needed quick action as there was a problem
The low haemoglobin, and the lower blood pressure, was a sign of an internal bleeding problem
A referral to the hospital was made urgent to see a specialist in case it was a more serious problem

Detailed checks of blood and an examination called Gastroscopy and Colonoscopy was ordered
I was lucky to secure a rapid Gastroscopy* and Colonoscopy* appointment that was ordered
No problem with the Colonoscopy but the Gastroscopy showed a growth with health hazard
A CT* scan was ordered to confirm and identify of the growth that posed as a potential health hazard

The CT scan indicated a T3* growth of abnormal cells that raised the suspicion of a cancer
The position and the rate of growth did not warrant a confirmation of cancer
Staging Laparoscopy* and Gastroscopy were ordered to reaffirm if the growth was a cancer
The conclusion that it was a GIST*, a rare type cist, later classed as a cancer was the answer

The PET* scan that was ordered was to confirm the GIST size and mode of treatment
I was weak, tired, worried after the above ordeal but there was the question of options of treatment
The consultant, who was calm and reassuring, led me to take keyhole surgery as treatment
Laparoscopic Excision of the GIST was the operation, the mode most appropriate for treatment

I woke up in the recovery room after the operation with wires and tubes that checked life vitals

In ward 727 I was cared for by dedicated nurses who constantly checked the life vitals

In a room of four I could see others suffering and pain, I remain calm as my pain was minimal

On day four, with no tubes and wires the Doctor hinted that I could go home, I felt normal

Reflecting on life I was glad I followed the treatment that helped in the removal of the GIST

At home in good progress in the healing process, I thought of life after and without the GIST

With an improving health one wonders what each passing year will offer without the GIST

I felt happy, relaxed and thankful to all who searched, detected, found and removed the GIST

MEDICAL TERMINOLOGY
USED ABOVE

Partial thyroidectomy—*when one side of the gland in front of the neck is removed surgically due to swelling or disease*

GIST*—*Gastro Intestinal Stromal Tumour, is a rare slow growth cancer of the GI tract*

CT*-*Computed Tomography, utilises X-rays to produce pictures showing the density of different organs in the body.*

T3*—*Staging describes the extent or severity of a person's cancer. Knowing the stage of disease helps the doctor plan treatment and estimates the person's prognosis. T1, T2, T3, T4; indicate the size and or the extent of the primary tumour*

Gastroscopy*—*A gastroscopy is a medical procedure during which a thin, flexible tube called an endoscope is used to look inside the stomach. It is also known as an endoscopy.*

Colonoscopy*—*is an endoscopic examination of the large bowel and the distal part of the small bowel by a flexible camera passed though the anus*

Staging Laparoscopy*—*is a keyhole surgery under a general anaesthetic that allows the surgeon to insert a camera into the abdomen to view the major internal organs, helping to look at the surface of the liver, bowels and other organs to check for spread of disease.*

PET*—*Positron Emission Tomography, this is an imaging technique which uses a small amount of radioactive tracer, a product similar to sugar (18Fluorodeoxyglucose) The images produced show how the body is functioning.*

A visit to the memory lane:

The thought of travelling along the winding dusty road to Nanjara was never the same as the memory of such close departed friends and relatives made Touwa get a feeling of sadness loneliness and a little insecure as he realised that the gift of life can be short lived. That journey was significant as Touwa was invited to celebrate the lives of the departed namely the ten years after the death of Salema,

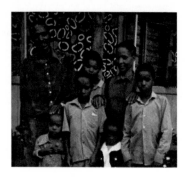

Thadeus family2

Salimu, Shenji and uncle Mkosi. The celebration was termed 'Salema's memorial'.

The flight to Dar es Salaam took Dorisi, Hagali and Touwa who were received by Ndesumbuka. It was the first time Hagali saw his father's Dar es Salaam house. It was also a first time he met so many cousins, the Kimarios, the Mrosos, the Tarimos, the Silayos and many more from the expansion of the Salema family. The arranged transport carried most of the family from Mbezi towards Moshi town and eventually to

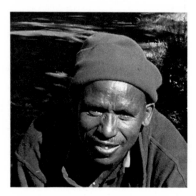

Failosi

234

Nanjara. Unlike the old days the road towards Moshi town was smooth with few potholes, enabling a speedy travel. The formerly 12 hour journeys took eight hours to Nanjara. The road towards Nanjara was no longer narrow, twisting or dusty meandering road but a fairly straight, smooth (macadamised)road enabling the journey to be less tiresome. There were pylons carrying electric power all he way along the new road. There were bridges, wider and more secure. There were pipes that distributed water near the dwellings. There were better houses that replaced the huts. The youngest brother Tabuni and his family received the guests for the start of the great celebrations for the life of the late Salema. It was also the great moment for Touwa to meet the Nanjara folk, notable was Failosi and Arobo with his wife

Benadina and a friend, Makereti who never left the village. A new project in the village was noted. It was a bridge to cross river Tarakea at the area where Touwa and friends used to take stark naked swimming sessions. The project was reputed to have saved many lives as the river which was a dry bed most times could have sudden fast flowing stone carrying water in moments when rains fall in the mountain.

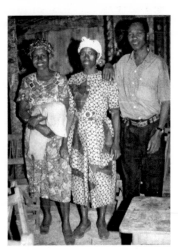

Arobo

The **22** children, the **99** grandchildren, the **55** great grandchildren, the possibility of a number of great-great grandchildren together with the village folk who knew him when he was alive were joined by those who did not know him in remembering Salema. They recalled his wit and humour, his jokes, his sentiments, his thoughts, his laughter and his good, bad and possibly humane acts, to mention few of what made him so loved during the celebration of his life. The meeting of such magnitude was a rare event but was loved by all. The celebration started with *'mbege'*, beers, 'kangara', *'busa'*—maize based alcoholic drink, soft drinks like orangeade, lemonade, soda water, and cola including many fruit juices. It was midday on the 15th day of September 2012 when the drinking started, while concurrently a selected and trusted few were busy slaughtering and eventually roasting and preparing the feast food. Some women were busy peeling bananas to be cooked with the meat of the cow that was slaughtered. The congregation was not a small group it included all Salema children, grands and great grands as the numbers shown above. In addition there were neighbours, friend of the family and do not forget cousins, nephews and nieces from Salema's sister and brother. Those who heard of the party but did not know the purpose of it, were also welcome. Last but not least friends of friends were also welcome. During the drinking through to eating, talking among groups and friends, introductions, laughter and cheer were the main activities broken by a speech or two to outline the purpose of the gathering. As the evening approached, a log fire was lit but the singing was missing. The younger folk had forgotten the tradition of singing and the words of the songs. The news from the radio and occasional music was the only songs that were heard.

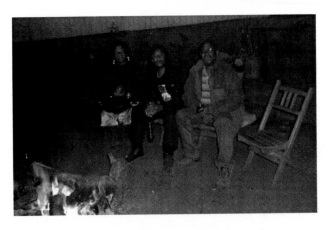

Log fire enjoyment

It was sad for Touwa to see that change.

Touwa however noted story telling and some comic hilarious jokes that made sitting by the log fire a pleasure that lasted till the early hours of the morning or when the *'mbege'* was finished without a hint of boredom. When the day came to pass, on reflection Touwa, Dorisi and Hagali all agreed it was a good way of

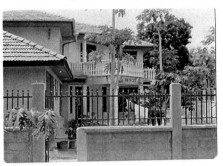

New mbezi house

remembering the life of a parent, a friend or a loved one. Small gatherings at Mashaka, Tabu and Tabuni that involved slaughter of goats, concluded the huge celebration that remembered the passing of Salema

The fourth morning after the numerous hand shakes and good bye, the journey to Moshi and Dar es Salaam started. Hagali made a glimpse of Touwa's lower primary school and remembered visiting it when he was 13 years old.

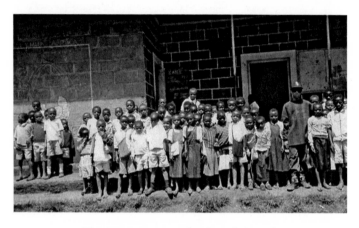

Nanjara primary school with Hagali

The journey to Dar es Salaam was concluded with a tour to Selous Game reserve that made the eventual flight to Birmingham an enjoyment worth remembering. In Dar es Salaam, Hagali explored the Mbezi village in real to reinforce the knowledge of the village studied from Google maps. He also explored the details of his father's new house in Mbezi, in order to relate to his brother, sister and the grandchildren. It was after arriving at home in Birmingham, that Touwa sat by the window one cold evening, enjoying a rare winter sunset in Birmingham that looked like a forest fire. It was at that time when reminiscing, that he remembered the unique sunset of Nanjara when the sun sets between the two peaks of Mount Kilimanjaro and how the road was no longer dusty and meandering. It was also at that time he remembered the progress some family members

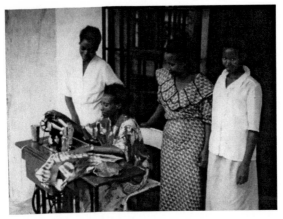

Mary a sister Sewing and teaching

had achieved through his ideological or material help, while reflecting on the significance of the Nanjara style party. He

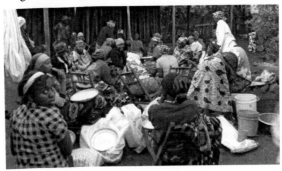

'Preparations for the great party'

switched his thought to the future, hoped to have a good life like Salema, and looked forward to his retirement that was soon to be eminent.

The Salema lineage

A brief history of Salema's origins:

The great Bantu migration that moved southwards forming the currently known 140 ethnic groups like the Chagga, Kikuyu, Luhya, Shona, Sukuma, Haya, Baganda, in the Congo, Lingala and far south as the Zulu. The Chagga ethnic group was formed in about 1000 to 1500 AD when it moved and settled around Mount Kilimanjaro. To do that settlement they had to drive off Pigmies and the Wangassa who occupied the mountain slopes.

According to Musee son of Katarimo, the forefathers of Salema were from Ngaseni, a land between the streams of Mashima and Ngolulwe in Usseri that was a home for the Ngaza people. The Ngaza people were said to migrate from the north, lands close to the current Middle East that may include Israel or Palestine. A large group consisting of men and women travelled southwards to take the body of their dead Queen who before her death wanted to be laid to rest on the slopes of Mount Kilimanjaro. After the body was laid to rest into a crater that also served as an elephant grave, the group found that the land was rich in abundance of food and decided to settle. Although many of the Ngaza were driven away by the encroaching Chagga people, some like those who settled in Usseri were not found until they had developed a language and culture different to that of the Usseri people.

Nakovisi and his first wife Masuai Furanii had three children namely Katarimo, Shenji (Kahumba)and a girl named Maruwa. They were all living in Ngaseni and spoke the dialect of Wangasa. Shenji married to Yohana Mamnana (From the Matimira family)and had two sons Mkosi and Salema and a girl, Rosalia. The children of Shenji spoke less of Ngasa dialect and more of the Chagga dialect. Salema's auntie Maruwa was captured in the Masai-Chagga war, and moved to Masai. Another war by a group from Arusha again captured Maruwa and moved her to Arusha where she had two children. When the Chagga from Kibongoto defeated Arusha, Maruwa was captured again and was sent to Kibongoto where she was accidentally discovered by traders who were friends of Shenji. A brief union of Shenji and his sister helped him to secure his dowry, a cow he named "*manembara*" that produced many offspring. At Kibongoto a region on the Western slopes of Kilimanjaro, Maruwa got a son and called him Mseri. It was the son of Mseri (a grandchild of Maruwa)that was discovered by Musee son of Katarimo in the later years that led to the story of Maruwa being known. Nakovisi had other wives and children like Matembea, Saroni Yeronimi, Tomaa, Inyasi, Teresia, Sesilia and Victoria who have played their role in the families that occupy many of the villages in the slopes of Mount Kilimanjaro.

-*END*-

Appendix:
Salema lineage 2012

THE SALEMA FAMILY LINEAGE

00	Shenji, his 3 Wives and children (Salema' parents)			
Anthony Kahumba Nakovisi Silayo (1870-1978)	Yohana Mamnana (1899-1974)	Martini Mkosi Kimario (1915-2005)	Vincent Salema Kimario (1921-2003)	Rosalia Makimario (1922-1997)
	Mamucholo Mshiki (1909-1997)	Sumaili Silayo	Kimwai (Triphone) Tarimo	Failosi Mrema	Benadina Mamrema
	Maktasi Kabumba (1920-1957)	Katarina Maswai		

0	Vincent Salema The three wives and children (Generation 1)								
Vincent Salema Kimario (1921-2002)	Josephine Mkasumaiti Mamroso (1921-1959)	1-Marceli Salimu Silayo (1943-2007)	2-Theresi Mkaleso Makimario 1945-	3-Paul Touwa Mroso 1949-	4-Matei Ndesumbuka Kimario 1951-	5-Fransi Melikoi Mroso 1953-	6-Daniel Tabuni Kimario 1955-	7-Tadei Tabu Kimario (Kimbulumbulu) 1957-	8-*Mashaka Josephat Vincent 1954-
	Alina Mkasalia Matesha 1924-	9-Victoria Mkabasia 1952-	10-Andrea Yonaa Silayo 1954-	11-Eugenia Mamkwe 1957-	12-Dismasi Mkwe Kimario 1961-	13-Meresiana Mshiki 1964-	14-Gaspari Mkosi Kimario 1967-		
	Mamoroi Elizabeth Salema (1942-1986)	15-Yohana Mamnana 1960-	16-Fortunata Mamkwe 1962-	17-Rosalia Mshiki 1964-	18-Anthony Kahumba Kimario 1966-	19-Edita Makimario 1968-	20-Adriani Tete Sinare 1972-	21-Ziporah Makinavei Salema 1974-	22-Martin Nakuvesia Kimario (Kinyeti) 1978-

Salema's Children and their children (Salema's Grandchildren(Generation 2)

	Salema Family	Wife/husb	a-Josephine Mkasumaili	b-Oliver Mamkwe	c-Demenria Manyengela	d-Pricilla Marceli Masilayo	e-Vincent Marceli Salema	f-Dorisi Marceli Mkaleso	g-Novati marceli Matolo	h-Priva Marceli Mroso	i-Nimta Mshiki Bahati
1	Marceli Salimu Silayo	Olympia Mkasara mamasawe	a-Josephine Mkasumaili	b-Oliver Mamkwe	c-Demenria Manyengela	d-Pricilla Marceli Masilayo	e-Vincent Marceli Salema	f-Dorisi Marceli Mkaleso	g-Novati marceli Matolo	h-Priva Marceli Mroso	i-Nimta Mshiki Bahati
		*Girlfriend	j-Desideri ** Marceli Silayo								
2	Theresia Mkaleso	Didas Kiberenge Terimo	a-Chistina Didas Matarimo	b-Gaudensi Kiberenge	c-Josephine Mkasumaili	d-Ginsela Mshiki	e-Vincent Didas Salema	f-Steven Silayo	g-Marceli didas Salimu	h-Zenobia Mkabasia	
3	Paul Touwa Mroso	Dora Peter York	a-Heidi Paula Mroso(Mkasu)	b-Anthony Paul Mroso (Hagali)	c-Steven Paul Mroso (Siti)						
4	Matei Ndesumbuka	Simforasa Peter	a-Happiness Mkasumaili	b-Emanuelle Salema	c-Hellena Mamkwe	d-Julieth mkaleso	e-*Zainabu Sivangi				
5	Francis Melikoi Mroso	Raheli Pima	a-Josephine Francis Mroso	b-Patrick Francis Mroso	C0Jackson Francis Mroso	e-Anna Francis Mroso	f-Ernest Francis Mroso				

#										
6	**Daniel lenkoya Kimario**	**Pauline Kavengi**	a-Peter Salema	b-Josephine Tosi	c-David Ketukei	d-James Lenkoya	e-Elijah lemaiyan			
7	**Thadeus Tabuni Kimbulumbulu**	**Bernadette Mamroso**	a-Vincent Thadeus Salema	b-Josephine Mkasumaili	c-Anna Mkadabu	e-James Dobi	f-Marceli Thadeus Salimu	g-George Mbeya	h-Julieth Mshiki	i-Primus Touwa
8	**Mashaka Josephat vincent**	**Mary Mamroso**	a-Magdaline Shija	b-John Kashije						

9	Victoria Mkabasia	Paul Msafiri (Mamkoku)	a-Alina Mamkwe	b-Airin Mshiki	c-Eric Ngeleshi	d-Josephine Mkwe Sereha	e-Orest Tesha	f-Arikadi Oiso	g-Melkiory Terimo	h-Julius Andrea	i-Jenofer Andrea
10	Andrea Yonaa Silayo	Epifania Mkanusu	a-Alina matesha	b-Vincent Salema (Jangi)	c-Mary Masilayo						
11	Eugenia Mamkwe	Richard Tarimo	a-Prakseda Makanje	b-Edgar Salakana	c-Anselimu Salema	d-Lilian Matesha	e-Rosemina Mshiki	f-Sara Masilayo			
12	Dismasi Mkwe Kimario	Devota Mashayo	a-Gastone Salema	b-Goodwin mkwe	c-Elizabeth Mkasalia	d-Avit silayo					
13	Meresiana Mshiki	Akley Salimu	a-Lucia Masalema	b-Emiliana kosma							
14	Gaspari Mkosi Kimario	Virginia Masilemu	a-Lilian Matesha	b-Vincent Gaspar Salema							
15	Yohana Mamnana	Charles kishinda	a-Amadeus Teri	b-Arkadi kimario	c-Digna Mamrina	d-Elizabeth Makavishe	e-Lucia Charles	f-Sidora Charles			
16	Fortunata Mamkwe	Eldergardes Kanje	a-Josephat Kanje	b-Bernadina Mamasawe	c-Vincent Kimario		e-Gaudiosa Mshiki				
17	Rosalia Mshiki	-	a-Duncan Mboshe	b-Joyce Mwandomi	c-Eunice Nyabeta	d-Rukia Mshiki	e-Supa				
18	Anthony Kahumba Kimario	Elizabeth Mkabeti	a-Elizabeth Mamoroi	b-Kevin tumaini Kahumba	c-Purity Mamkwe	d-Paul Junior	e-Eric Mushi				

19	Edita Makimario	Ramadhani Loya waziri	a-Aisha Ramadhani	
20	Adriani Tete Sinare	Happiness Adriani	a-Josephine Adriani	b-Neema adriani
21	Ziporah Makinavei Salema	George Sande	a-Jubilant Mungai	b-Janet b-Nyakio
22	Martin Nakovisi Kimario Kinyeti)	Theresia John Kimario	a- Gladness Martine	b- Godliven Martine

	Salema Family	Wife/husband				
			Salema grandchildren's children (Great Grandchildren) Generation 3			
1a	Josephine Mkasumaili	Karoli Shayo	1-Veronica Mkahimo	2-Libberia Mkasara	3-Agnes Mshiki	4-Winifrida Mamkwe
1b	Oliver Mamkwe	Harry C M Sabbas	1-Sabas Mshikamano	2-Dickson stambuli	3-gloria sheila	
1c	Dementria manyengela	Arbogast Tarimo	1-Gloria Tarimo	2-Gilda Tarimo	3-Gemma Tarimo	4-Gudila Tarimo
1d	Pricilla Marceli Masilayo	Andrea Rotas Silayo	1-Happiness Silayo	2-Gifti Silayo		
1e	Vincent Marceli Salema	*				
1f	Dorisi Marceli Mkaleso	Amani	1- Abel	2- Alvin		
1g	Novati marceli matolo	*				
1h	Priva Marceli Mroso	*				
1i	Nimta Mshiki Bahati	*				
1j	Desideri Marceli Silayo	Fides Desideri	1-Priscus Silayo	2-calvin silayo		
2a	Chistina Didas Matarimo	Firmini Matei	1-Veronica Firmini	2-Staton Firmini	3-Theresia firmini	
2b	Gaudensi Kiberenge	Lucia Tarimo	1-Didas Tarimo	2-Gaspar Tarimo	3-Vincent Tarimo	
2c	Josephine Mkasumaili	Marki	1-Janet Marki	2-Theresia marki		
2d	Ginsela Mshiki	Musee Matei	1-Emanuel Musee	2-Analia musee	3-Didas Musee	
2e	Vincent Didas Salema	Sefera Mashirima				
2f	Steven Silayo	*				
2g	Marceli didas Salimu	*	1- Sedrick Marceli (Twins)	2- Sedrina Marceli (Twins)		

249

2h	Zenobia Mkabasia	John	1- Gladness			
3a	**Heidi Paula Mroso(Mkasu)**	**Y Bowers**	1-Junaide bowers	2-Unaysaah McDowell	3-Amarah Hector	4-Rayaan Hector
3b	**Anthony Paul Mroso (Hagali)**	**Donita Deana Forde**	1-Kiambu AnthonyMroso	2-Kai Anthony Mroso	3-Rowan Anthony Mroso	
3c	**Steven Paul Mroso (Siti)**	*	1- Renee A Mroso			
4a	**Happiness Mkasumaili**	**Aristid Kanje**	1-Irene Kanje			
4b	**Emanuelle Salema**	*				
4c	**Hellena Mamkwe**	*				
4d	**Julieth Mkaleso**	*				
4e	***Zainabu Sewangi**	**Gady**	1- Mugisha	2- Gloria Gady		
5a	Josephine Francis Mroso	*				
5b	Patrick Francis Mroso	*				
5c	Jackson Francis Mroso	*	1-Ebenezar Jackson Mrosso			
5d	Anna Francis Mroso	**Nicodemas Mushi**				
5e	Ernest Francis Mroso	*				
6a	Vincent Daniel Salema	*				
6b	Josephine Mato (Tosi)	*				
6c	David Kitukei	*				
6d	James Lenkoya	*				
7a	Vincent thadeus Salema	**Selista Vicent**	1-Brillian			
7b	Josephine Mkasumaili	**Anicet Vicent**	1-Michelle Anicet	2-Michael Anicet	3-Myleen Anicet	
7c	Anna mkadabu	*	1-Victor	2-Joyleen		

7d	James Dobi	*		
7e	Marceli thadeus Salimu	*		
7f	George Mbeya	*		
8a	Magdaline Shija			
8b	John Kashije	*		
9a	Alina Mamkwe	**Timothy Castro**	1-Suzzy mary	
9b	Airin Mshiki	*		
9c	Eric Ngeles	*		
10a	Alina matesha	*		
10b	Vincent Salema (Jangi)	**Severa Coleman**	1- Epiphania Mkanusu	2-Denis Kimario

10c	Mary Masilayo	*	1-Bassy Masilayo
10d	Josephine Mkwe Sereha	*	
10e	Orest Tesha	*	
10f	Arikadi Oiso	*	
10g	Melkiory Terimo	*	
10h	Julius Andrea	*	
10i	Jenifer Andrea	*	
11a	Prakseda Makanje		
11b	Edgar Salakana		
11c	Anselimu Salema		
11d	Lilian Matesha		
11e	Rosemina Mshiki		
11f	Sara Masilayo		
12a	Gastone Salema		
12b	Goodwin mkwe		
12c	Elizabeth Mkasalia		
12d	Avit silayo		
13a	Lucia Masalema		
13b	Emiliana kosma		
14a	Lilian Matesha		
14b	Vincent Gaspar Salema		
15a	Amadeus Teri		
15b	Arkardi kimario		
15c	Digna Mamrina		
15d	Elizabeth Makavishe		
15e	Lucia Charles		
15f	Sidora Charles		
16a	Josephat Kanje		
16b	Bernadina Mamasawe		
16c	Vincent Kimario		
16d	Gaudiosa Mshiki		
17a	Duncan Mboshe		
17b	Joyce Mwandomi		
17c	Eunice Nyabeta		
17d	Rukia Mshiki		

17e	Supa	
18a	Elizabeth Mamoroi	
18b	Kevin Tumaini Kahumba	
18c	Purity Mamkwe	
18d	Paul Junior	
18e	Eric Mushi	
19a	Aisha Ramadhani	
20a	Josephine Adriani	
20b	Neem a adriani	
21a	Jubilant J Mungai	
21b	Janet Nyakio	
22a	*	

Salema's Great Grandchildren's Children (Great-Great Grandchildren)_- Generation 4		
	Salema Family	**Wife/husband**
1a1	Veronica Mkahimo	
1a2	Libberia Mkasara	
1a3	Agnes Mshiki	
1a4	Winifrida Mamkwe	
2a1	1-Sabas Mshikamano	
1a2	2-Dickson stambuli	
1a3	3-gloria sheila	
1b1	Gloria Tarimo	
1b2	Gilda Tarimo	
1b3	Gemma Tarimo	
1b4	Gudila Tarimo	
1c1	Happiness Silayo	
1c2	-Gifti Silayo	
1d1	Emanuel Musee	
1d2	Analia musee	
1d3	Didas Musee	
1j1	Priscus Silayo	
1j2	calvin silayo	

2a1	Veronica Firmini		
2a2	Staton Firmini		
2a3	Theresia firmini		
2b1	Didas Tarimo		
2b2	Gaspar Tarimo		
2b3	Vincent Tarimo		
2c1	Janet Marki		
2c2	Theresia marki		
2d1	Emanuel Musee		
2d2	Analia musee		
2d3	Didas Musee		
2e1	*		
3a1	Junaide bowers		
3a2	Unaysaah McDowel		
3a3	Amarah Hector		
3a4	Rayaan Hector		
3b1	-Kiambu Anthony Mroso		
3b2	-Kai Anthony Mroso		
3b3	Rowan Anthony Mroso		
3c1	Renee A Mroso		
*			
9a1	Suzzy mary		
*			
10b1	Epiphania Mkanusu		
10b2	Denis Kimario		
10c1	Bassy Masilayo		